# CO-OCCURRING MENTAL ILLNESS
## and
# SUBSTANCE USE DISORDERS

## A Guide to Diagnosis and Treatment

# CO-OCCURRING MENTAL ILLNESS
## and
# SUBSTANCE USE DISORDERS

## A Guide to Diagnosis and Treatment

*Edited by*

Jonathan D. Avery, M.D.
John W. Barnhill, M.D.

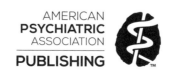

AMERICAN
**PSYCHIATRIC**
ASSOCIATION
**PUBLISHING**

If you wish to buy 50 or more copies of the same title, please go to www.appi.org/specialdiscounts for more information.

Copyright © 2018 American Psychiatric Association Publishing

ALL RIGHTS RESERVED

First Edition

Manufactured in the United States of America on acid-free paper
21  20          5  4  3  2

American Psychiatric Association Publishing
1000 Wilson Boulevard
Arlington, VA 22209-3901
www.appi.org

**Library of Congress Cataloging-in-Publication Data**
Names: Avery, Jonathan D., editor. | Barnhill, John W. (John Warren), editor. | American Psychiatric Publishing, publisher.
Title: Co-occurring mental illness and substance use disorders : a guide to diagnosis and treatment / edited by Jonathan D. Avery, John W. Barnhill.
Description: First edition. | Arlington, Virginia : American Psychiatric Association Publishing, [2018] | Includes bibliographical references and index.
Identifiers: LCCN 2017030620 (print) | LCCN 2017031909 (ebook) | ISBN 9781615371594 (ebook) | ISBN 9781615370559 (pbk. : alk. paper)
Subjects: | MESH: Diagnosis, Dual (Psychiatry) | Mental Disorders—diagnosis | Substance-Related Disorders—diagnosis | Mental Disorders—therapy | Substance-Related Disorders—therapy | Problems and Exercises
Classification: LCC RC473.D54 (ebook) | LCC RC473.D54 (print) | NLM WM 18.2 | DDC 616.89/075—dc23
LC record available at https://lccn.loc.gov/2017030620

**British Library Cataloguing in Publication Data**
A CIP record is available from the British Library.

# CONTENTS

## PART 1
### *THE INITIAL INTERVIEW AND COMPREHENSIVE ASSESSMENT*

## PART 2
### *CO-OCCURRING DISORDERS*

# CONTRIBUTORS

**Luke J. Archibald, M.D.**
Clinical Assistant Professor of Psychiatry, NYU School of Medicine, New York

**Evelyn Attia, M.D.**
Professor of Clinical Psychiatry, Weill Cornell Medical College, White Plains, New York; Clinical Professor of Psychiatry, Columbia University College of Physicians and Surgeons, New York, New York

**Jonathan D. Avery, M.D.**
Assistant Clinical Professor of Psychiatry, Assistant Dean of Student Affairs, Weill Cornell Medical College; Assistant Attending Psychiatrist, New York-Presbyterian Hospital, Payne Whitney Clinic, New York, New York

**Maria Andrea Baez, M.D.**
Clinical Assistant Professor of Psychiatry, New York University School of Medicine, New York, New York

**John W. Barnhill, M.D.**
Professor of Clinical Psychiatry, DeWitt Wallace Senior Scholar, and Vice Chair for Psychosomatic Medicine, Department of Psychiatry, Weill Cornell Medical College; Chief, Consultation-Liaison Service, New York-Presbyterian Hospital, Weill Cornell Medical Center Hospital for Special Surgery, New York, New York

**Sonal Batra, M.D.**
Fellow, Pharmaceutical Medicine, Rutgers Robert Wood Johnson Medical School, Piscataway, New Jersey

**Shannon G. Caspersen, M.D., M.Phil.**

Clinical Instructor, Weill Cornell Medical College, New York-Presbyterian Hospital, New York, New York

**Silvia Franco, M.D.**

Psychiatry Resident, The Icahn School of Medicine at Mount Sinai/St. Luke's–Roosevelt Hospital Psychiatry Program, New York, New York

**Bernadine H. Han, M.D., M.S.**

Resident, Payne-Whitney Psychiatry, Weill Cornell Medicine/New York-Presbyterian Hospital, New York, New York

**Grace Hennessy, M.D.**

Clinical Assistant Professor of Psychiatry, New York University School of Medicine; Director, Substance Abuse Recovery Program, Department of Veterans Affairs, New York Harbor Healthcare System, New York Campus, New York, New York

**Rocco A. Iannucci, M.D.**

Instructor in Psychiatry, Harvard Medical School, Boston, Massachusetts; Director, McLean Fernside, Princeton, Massachusetts

**Sean P. Kerrigan, M.D.**

Assistant Professor of Psychiatry, Weill Cornell Medical College, New York-Presbyterian Hospital, White Plains, New York

**Zain Khalid, M.D.**

PGY-2 Resident, Department of Psychiatry, Rutgers New Jersey Medical School, Newark, New Jersey

**Ariel Kor, Ph.D.**

Department of Counseling and Clinical Psychology, Teachers College, Columbia University, New York, New York

**Frances R. Levin, M.D.**

Kennedy-Leavy Professor of Psychiatry; Director, Division on Substance Abuse, Department of Psychiatry, Columbia University, New York, New York

**Sean X. Luo, M.D., Ph.D.**

Leon Levy Fellow, Department of Psychiatry, Columbia University, New York, New York

**Steve Martino, Ph.D.**
Professor of Psychiatry, Yale University School of Medicine, New Haven, Connecticut; Chief, Psychology Service, VA Connecticut Healthcare System, West Haven, Connecticut

**Rebecca A. Nejat, M.D.**
Chief Resident, Weill Cornell Department of Psychiatry, New York, New York

**Mayumi Okuda, M.D.**
Director, Gambling Disorders Clinic, Department of Psychiatry, New York State Psychiatric Institute/Columbia University, New York, New York

**David T. Pilkey, Ph.D.**
Assistant Professor of Psychiatry, Yale University School of Medicine, New Haven, Connecticut; Program Manager, Substance Abuse Day Program, VA Connecticut Healthcare System, West Haven, Connecticut

**Richard K. Ries, M.D.**
Professor, Department of Psychiatry and Behavioral Sciences, University of Washington, Seattle, Washington

**Caitlin Snow, M.D.**
Assistant Professor of Clinical Psychiatry, New York-Presbyterian/ Weill Cornell Medicine, New York, New York

**Howard R. Steinberg, Ph.D.**
Assistant Professor of Psychiatry, Yale University School of Medicine, New Haven, Connecticut; Program Manager, Psychosocial Residential Rehabilitation Treatment Program, VA Connecticut Healthcare System, West Haven, Connecticut

**J. David Stiffler, M.D.**
Clinical Assistant Professor of Psychiatry, New York University School of Medicine; Medical Director, The Steven A. Cohen Military Family Clinic, New York, New York

**Lauren Stossel, M.D.**
Forensic Psychiatry Fellow, New York University, New York, New York

**Roger D. Weiss, M.D.**
Professor of Psychiatry, Harvard Medical School, Boston, Massachusetts; Chief, Division of Alcohol and Drug Abuse, McLean Hospital, Belmont, Massachusetts

**Eric Yarbrough, M.D.**

Director of Psychiatry, Callen-Lorde Community Health Center, New York, New York; President, The Association of LGBTQ Psychiatrists, Philadelphia, Pennsylvania

**Christine Yuodelis-Flores, M.D.**

Associate Professor, Department of Psychiatry and Behavioral Sciences, University of Washington, Seattle, Washington

**Erin Zerbo, M.D.**

Assistant Professor, Department of Psychiatry, Rutgers New Jersey Medical School, Newark, New Jersey

## Disclosure of Competing Interests

*The following contributors to this book have indicated a financial interest in or other affiliation with a commercial supporter, a manufacturer of a commercial product, a provider of a commercial service, a nongovernmental organization, and/or a government agency, as listed below:*

**Frances R. Levin, M.D.**—Dr. Levin received medication from U.S. World-Med for this trial and served as a consultant to GW Pharmaceuticals and Eli Lily, and served on an advisory board to Shire in 2006–2007. Dr. Levin also serves as a consultant to Major League Baseball regarding the diagnosis and treatment of ADHD.

*The following contributors to this book have reported no competing interests during the year preceding manuscript submission:*

Luke J. Archibald, M.D.
Jonathan D. Avery, M.D.
Maria Andrea Baez, M.D.
John W. Barnhill, M.D.
Shannon G. Caspersen, M.D., M.Phil.
Silvia Franco, M.D.
Bernadine H. Han, M.D., M.S.
Rocco A. Iannucci, M.D.
Sean P. Kerrigan, M.D.
Zain Khalid, M.D.
Ariel Kor, Ph.D.

Sean X. Luo, M.D., Ph.D.
Steve Martino, Ph.D.
Rebecca A. Nejat, M.D.
Mayumi Okuda, M.D.
David T. Pilkey, Ph.D.
Richard K. Ries, M.D.
Howard R. Steinberg, Ph.D.
J. David Stiffler, M.D.
Lauren Stossel, M.D.
Eric Yarbrough, M.D.
Christine Yuodelis-Flores, M.D.
Erin Zerbo, M.D.

# INTRODUCTION

*Co-occurring Mental Illness and Substance Use Disorders: A Guide to Diagnosis and Treatment* is an evidence-based approach to people with at least two psychiatric disorders, one of which relates to substance use. This population of patients was formerly known as having a "dual diagnosis." Our primary goal is to provide the clinician with a straightforward approach to people with complicated presentations. Each chapter is based on a specific case that is written in such a way as to highlight generalizable suggestions. Our strongest central recommendation is simple: people should be tactfully but persistently evaluated for a broad range of co-occurring disorders, and then each of these disorders should be given clinical attention. At times, treatment for a particular disorder can be deferred, but for most co-occurring disorders, therapeutic success is much more likely if treatment is integrated, based on evidence, and focused on all relevant diagnoses.

Within psychiatry, co-occurring disorders are more the rule than the exception. People with substance use disorders typically have at least one co-occurring psychiatric disorder, while people with a primary psychiatric disorder often have at least one co-occurring substance use disorder. When there are two co-occurring disorders, there are often several others.

Substances of abuse have a complex relationship with mood, behavior, memory, and all the variables that go into making us human. It can be challenging to determine whether the presentation (e.g., depression, mania, confusion) is a manifestation of a primary psychiatric disorder or of substance intoxication, withdrawal, or chronic use. Further, people with co-occurring disorders often have complex psychosocial situations, complicated histories, and a seemingly entrenched pattern of failed treatments. Given the number of psychiatric disorders and the number of substances of abuse, the potential clinical complexity can feel overwhelming to clinicians, families, and patients. Fortunately, there are straightforward approaches to this complexity.

Let's consider a difficult but fairly routine case of co-occurring disorders. David is a 19-year-old man who presents for an evaluation after being arrested for selling MDMA (ecstasy) at a rave party. His affluent parents were able to get the criminal charges dropped, but they desperately want help for their son. David has been smoking marijuana almost daily since age 12 and has, in recent years, developed a daily habit of alternating cocaine and heroin in order to "fine tune" his mood. He sells ecstasy at rave parties in order to gain access to money, parties, drugs, and women. David has successfully taken amphetamine for his attention-deficit/hyperactivity disorder (ADHD) (combined presentation), which he, his parents, and his teachers agreed was helpful. A recent psychiatrist discontinued the amphetamine out of concern for abuse, though David insisted that he tended to be "short" on the amphetamine by the end of the month, not because he sells or over-uses, but because Sally, his 17-year-old sister, steals his supply. Sally had always been "perfect," but ever since a difficult breakup with a possibly abusive boyfriend, she has become moody and "way too skinny."

David, himself, attends classes at a local junior college. He made B's in high school but missed about half of the school days between ninth and twelfth grades so that he earned a GED rather than a high school diploma. David has briefly seen several psychotherapists, has recurrently tried 12-step programs, and has, in the past year, twice relapsed immediately after 30-day drug rehabs. David's parents are in the midst of a stormy divorce fueled by the father's persistent risk taking, irritability, and sexual indiscretions. The father averages a liter of vodka every 2 days, which he says is the only thing that can get him to sleep. David's mother is depressed and anxious and averages about 4 mg of clonazepam each day. David says he is a "clean needle fanatic" and insists that he will never get HIV, but he describes himself as a "nocturnal nihilist" with little hope that he'll live to reach age 21.

How best to approach David's complexity? One option is to identify a single problem as the focus for treatment. For example, David might be seen to have cocaine, heroin, and marijuana use disorders and be referred to either a 12-step program or a drug rehab. This approach has already failed multiple times, however, and so it might be useful to broaden the diagnostic possibilities to include undiagnosed and untreated depressive, anxiety, and/or insomnia disorder. The only co-occurring disorder that has received clinical attention appears to be ADHD, and a recent psychiatrist discontinued pharmacological treatment of the ADHD out of concern that the treatment (amphetamine) could be fueling his other substance use disorders. At this point, we would suggest that David needs attention paid to these co-occurring disorders if he is going to live successfully into adulthood. To help provide a clear but integrated plan, a clinician might read this book's chapters on ADHD, depression, anxiety, adolescence, and 12-step programs.

This book also features chapters on how to effectively work with disorders that might be affecting other members of David's family. For example, David's sister may be stealing his amphetamines, but she may have also developed an eating disorder, PTSD, and/or an anxiety or depressive disorder. David's mother appears to have depression, anxiety, and a benzodiazepine use disorder. His father might have an alcohol use disorder as well as a diagnosis on the bipolar spectrum. In each case, the likelihood of a successful outcome is enhanced if an integrated treatment plan is developed for their co-occurring disorders.

Before a treatment plan can be organized, however, it is necessary to identify the co-occurring disorders. Inaccurate or incomplete diagnoses will likely lead the treatment to founder, as will an insecure alliance. For that reason, the initial face-to-face sessions are especially important in this population. This book includes many tips on how to interview this group of patients, including entire chapters on motivational interviewing, the diagnostic assessment, and the initial interview.

Effective medications are available for both substance use disorders and co-occurring psychiatric disorders. Addiction specialists are generally aware of the strong evidence for medications that reduce craving, but they might be slow to pharmacologically treat the co-occurring disorders. General psychiatrists may be comfortable using medications to treat such disorders as depression or anxiety, but they may undervalue such medications as naltrexone and buprenorphine, which are generally effective and have few adverse effects. *Co-occurring Mental Illness and Substance Use Disorders: A Guide to Diagnosis and Treatment* will maintain a consistent point of view that medications for substance use disorders should be at least considered as part of an integrated treatment, as should more "standard" psychiatric medications.

This book is organized around 18 cases. The first two cases address interviewing and assessment. Each of the next eight cases focuses on a specific group of mental illness (e.g., depressive disorders, ADHD) and how to treat the mental illness and the substance use disorders that are highly comorbid with that illness. The subsequent four cases focus on specific treatments for co-occurring disorders. The final four cases focus on treating co-occurring disorders in special populations.

You have options in reading this casebook. You can read the 18 cases and discussions straight through. The cases do not depend on one another, however, and so you might start with a case that sounds interesting or about which you have a specific interest. The accompanying questions can be used to test your knowledge after you have read the chapter, though the questions can also be read prior to reading the chapter in order to help organize your reading. However it is used, we hope that this casebook can improve the experience of the clinicians who work with this population and improve the lives of the many people who suffer with these co-occurring disorders.

*Jonathan D. Avery, M.D.*
*John W. Barnhill, M.D.*

# PART 1

## THE INITIAL INTERVIEW AND COMPREHENSIVE ASSESSMENT

# THE INITIAL INTERVIEW

*John W. Barnhill, M.D.*

The core goals of the initial psychiatric evaluation are to ensure safety, understand the patient, and help develop a workable treatment plan. These straightforward principles are true for all patients, including people with co-occurring disorders. This chapter will address the structure of the initial interview and is intended to be digested alongside the book's other chapters, particularly the chapters on assessment (Chapter 2, "The Comprehensive Assessment") and motivational interviewing (Chapter 12, "Motivational Interviewing").

Most clinicians begin the initial interview by asking an open-ended question like "Tell me about what brought you here today." The initial question is followed by a period of active listening in which the interviewer demonstrates ongoing interest by asking questions such as "Tell me more about what you mean." This relatively unfocused phase of the interview gives the patient a chance to present his or her own concerns, which helps build an alliance and lays the groundwork for later treatment discussions. Open-ended questions also provide the interviewer with the opportunity to observe the patient and silently begin to make a set of tentative hypotheses.

| TABLE 1–1. | Physical symptoms that might point to substance use disorders |
|---|---|

Face: puffy, blushing, or pale

Poor overall health; runny nose; hacking cough

Poor hygiene

Unusual smells on breath, body, or clothes

Sweating

Cold palms

Tremor

Red, watery eyes

Pupils larger or smaller than usual

Needle marks

Poor physical coordination, stumbling gait

Altered activity and talkativeness

This early period of hypothesis generation is central to the evaluation of a patient who may have co-occurring disorders. Some patients present with a "loud" substance use disorder, but "quieter" diagnoses like anxiety or depression may be the bigger concern to the patient and may be obstacles to effective treatment. Other patients present without a substance use complaint but with a relatively obvious mood or anxiety disorder; this initial phase of the interview may provide clues to a "quiet" or hidden substance use disorder. In other words, the interview is an opportunity both to hear the "chief complaint" of the patient and to listen for what may not be clearly articulated.

Listening for what is *not* said is an interesting skill set that is part of becoming a clinician. In addition to the patient's actual words, the interviewer can learn from the "music" of the interview, such as the degree to which the interaction feels antagonistic, cooperative, or needy. This early phase of the interview is also an excellent time to tactfully observe physical signs that are often found in people with co-occurring disorders (Table 1–1).

This early phase of the evaluation can help interest the patient in his or her own problems. For example, the interviewer can ask, "Do you have thoughts as to why your wife might have called for your appointment?" or "Leaving aside what your husband wants for a moment, is there anything that is bothering you?" Genuine curiosity can help clarify the full range of problems and can also help develop the alliance that will be crucial to the treatment's eventual success.

This early phase of the interview is, thus, a time for the clinician to develop an alliance and begin to silently develop a differential diagnosis, a history of the present illness, and a mental status examination (MSE). A broad assessment effort is especially important in patients with co-occurring disorders, because evidence indicates that it is best to treat—or at least explicitly recognize—co-occurring disorders from the outset of the intervention.

Pressured for time, the busy clinician may decide to forgo this initial, open-ended phase in the pursuit of symptom clarification. Without a broad understanding of the patient's complaints, however, this clinician may develop a focused understanding of one aspect of the patient but miss other diagnoses as well as the patient's own concerns.

Although open-ended curiosity is generally the most effective initial strategy during this initial phase, some patients are unable to open up until asked some "warm-up" questions (e.g., demographic information). Still other patients are unable or unwilling to reveal sensitive information soon after meeting someone. Each interview is a bit different, and so the interviewer will likely have to remain flexible to be effective.

The later phase of the interview is focused on the interviewer's effort to convert the patient's story into the interviewer's own *history of the present illness* (HPI). This is an active process that requires the clinician to elicit and synthesize an assortment of patient behaviors and symptoms, bits of semi-reliable collateral information, possible comorbidities, unspoken hypotheses, prior (mis)diagnoses, and psychiatric, medical, social, family, and developmental histories.

Central to this reinterpretation of a patient's story into an HPI is the interviewer's ability to shift from a relatively open-ended "conversation" into more active, directive questioning. Interviewers make this transition in different ways, but it is often useful for the interviewer to directly indicate that he or she would like to pursue some specific details for a few minutes. This phase of data acquisition may involve a manualized assessment tool as described in Chapter 2, or it may be a more spontaneously intuitive process. Although the goal of the initial interview may be to arrive at a wonderfully robust three-dimensional picture of the patient, it can be helpful to recall that no initial interview is ever complete: additional information is likely to emerge as the relationship develops, as collateral information emerges, and as the patient's behaviors and symptoms evolve during the ensuing weeks and months. In other words, the interviewer need not feel pressured to completely "get" the patient during the initial interview.

For example, in Chapter 5 ("Posttraumatic Stress Disorder"), Joe presents with the problematic use of alcohol and marijuana. A former soldier, he is also suffering a variety of anxiety symptoms. When meeting a psychiatric interviewer for the first time, a patient like Joe might focus on substance abuse, or he might focus on anxiety or PTSD and insist that the alcohol and marijuana use is under control. Joe might also insist that he neither uses illicit drugs nor has a significant psychiatric issue; instead he might insist that his primary problem is an overly zealous wife who tricked him into the evaluation. The way Joe tells his story has implications in regard to understanding the patient and planning treatment options, but it is unlikely he will tell a completely thorough, historically accurate story.

Different listening styles bring their own strengths and potential weaknesses. For example, some excellent interviewers specifically target DSM-5 symptom clusters throughout much of the interview. If done in an unempathic way, however, excess focus on symptom lists can lead to a shortchanging of the alliance and diagnostic depth.

Others might interview based on what feels to them to be a small toolbox of therapeutic options, ready to bypass the diagnostic process in order to more efficiently recommend their preferred treatment. For example, a busy clinician might quickly assess a patient to have severe alcohol use disorder with a history of poor adherence to outpatient treatment programs. This can lead the clinician to short-circuit the assessment process once he or she recognizes that the treatment suggestion will ultimately be a half-hearted recommendation to Alcoholics Anonymous. Such a short-circuiting of the evaluation is likely to lead the clinician to miss co-occurring disorder(s) that could be contributing to the repeated treatment failures.

A more psychodynamically oriented therapist may listen primarily for unspoken psychological factors that contribute to psychiatric symptoms. For example, an initial psychodynamically oriented interview might yield a conclusion that unreliable early caregivers led the child to anger and frustration that could not be adequately expressed for fear of losing the parent's affection. This lifelong tendency may contribute to an adult patient's anxious and avoidant interactional style and medication nonadherence. At the same time, a co-occurring substance use or psychiatric disorder can, by itself, lead to significant anger, frustration, and nonadherence, regardless of underlying psychological issues. In other words, working within a psychodynamic model may lead to a stronger understanding of the person who has presented for help, but it can also lead to missing the substance abuse and psychiatric diagnoses.

Regardless of one's own theoretical tendency, it is generally wise to spend at least some time paying conscious attention to each aspect of the biopsychosocial framework. This can be especially helpful in patients whose most obvious psychiatric diagnosis is so loudly obvious that co-occurring disorders are ignored; recurrent treatment failures are often the result of inadequate attention being paid to relatively "quiet" co-occurring disorders. People with co-occurring disorders can also distract and frustrate their interviewers through a variety of typical distancing techniques. As is often the case in psychiatry, roadblocks can often be sidestepped if the interviewer remains patient, persistent, tactful, and curious (see Table 1–2 for examples).

A safety assessment is part of every initial psychiatric evaluation. In particular, we look for suicidality, homicidality, medical complications, and the likelihood of withdrawal from a substance. Safety information may come out naturally during the course of the interview, but it is generally wise to explicitly ask specifically about safety issues.

Most of the MSE can be assessed as part of the overall interview. The social, psychiatric, and developmental histories can help inform the diagnosis and treatment, while the history of prior substance abuse treatments can often be the single most useful piece of collateral information. It is difficult to know in advance when such information is going to be vital, and historical data can feel unimportant if not linked to the patient's presenting problem. Initial interviews conclude with a differential diagnosis and treatment plan, even if it is likely that both the diagnosis and the treatment are uncertain and likely to evolve with additional time.

The initial interview depends on a working knowledge of the fields of psychiatry and substance abuse. As is true for the fictional detective Sherlock Holmes, we are unlikely to notice pivotal details without a readily available knowledge base. As we listen, we silently consider, discard, and reconsider a large amount of information. These tentative assessments guide our interactions by helping us determine which issues should be more actively discussed and acted upon. Information acquisition can be felt as intrusive by the patient, but it can also be felt as supportive: clinicians who tactfully ask knowledgeable questions are implicitly communicating that they are genuinely interested and that they understand psychiatry, substance use, and people.

Given the ubiquity of online resources, it might not seem necessary to have a working knowledge of likely comorbidities, common symptom constellations, and treatment strategies. Although much can be gained by Internet access, it is unlikely that even the most dexterous interviewer can maintain eye contact with a patient while also trying to look things up online. Such preparation often begins with a regular practice of reading texts like this one. By helping to provide a framework for how to understand patients, such texts help inform the interview and help put other information into perspective.

---

**TABLE 1–2.  Typical comments that can de-skill an interviewer**

---

My drug use is no big deal.

I need ___ mg of my drug every 4 hours.

My situation is hopeless.

I can stop whenever I want.

Life is too boring without my drug.

All my friends use more than I do.

I don't know why my tox screen was positive—I don't take drugs.

As if you would understand.

---

For example, in Chapter 10 ("Gambling Disorder"), Peter is a long-time gambler who initially denied substance abuse. Given that about 75% of men with a gambling disorder also have an alcohol use disorder, the alert clinician might actively look for indications that Peter is not being entirely forthcoming when he denies a problem with alcohol. Such clues might include a withdrawal tremor, abnormal lab values, or collateral information.

While we observe the patient, the patient is sizing us up. Are we trustworthy, effective, and knowledgeable about the field? In regard to Peter, for example, the clinician who doggedly pursues an alcohol history may win that small piece of knowledge but lose the alliance. This may be a necessary price to pay to address safety concerns, but it may come with a cost to the alliance and eventual chances for treatment success. Concerns about the alliance need not lead the clinician to passivity, however, and it may be reasonable for the interviewer to simply say to Peter that alcohol use and gambling tend to co-occur. Such an assertion demonstrates the clinician's knowledge base and gives the patient a chance to elaborate on his earlier denial of an alcohol problem.

Three interacting philosophical notions tend to guide clinicians during the initial interview. Many clinicians were taught a "lean" approach to making a diagnosis. Sometimes called *Occam's razor*, or the law of diagnostic parsimony, this principle leads clinicians to search for the simplest explanation that can explain the clinical presentation. This principle has been balanced off by *Hickam's dictum*, which asserts that if patients have one disorder, they are likely to have more than one (this dictum is sometimes summarized as, "Patients can have as many diseases as they damn well please"). In other words, Hickam's dictum addresses our tendency to try to find a single diagnosis when multiple diagnoses are actively having an impact on one another. DSM-5 addresses this tendency by recommending that we identify pertinent diagnoses and generally not try to identify the single diagnosis that is the crucial, underlying precipitant of the patient's suffering.

A third philosophical notion is *Crabtree's bludgeon*, which posits that human imagination can create underlying theories about any unrelated bits of evidence. This assertion helps us slow down our tendency to prematurely identify a diagnosis and then search for supportive evidence while ignoring contradictory evidence. Taken together, these three principles can help the clinician make sense of information while avoiding the sorts of pitfalls that can bedevil any clinician. (For a further discussion of these principles, see Mani et al. 2011.)

Negotiation is an integral part of the evaluation process. Negotiation may take place at the end of the first session, or later, but treatments are likely to fail without the patient's participation. Negotiation might include the presentation of a diagnosis or differential diagnosis; psychoeducation; and exploration of treatment options. It can also be a good time to ask about patient satisfaction and the likelihood that the patient will participate in the recommended treatment. Exploration of these questions can determine treatment success.

The write-up plays an important role in the interview. For many interviewers, the cognitive process involved in writing helps clarify what can be a confusing amalgam of information. The writing process can also lead to a recognition that there are holes in the story that warrant follow-up questions. If so, the clinician should feel free to go back and get clarification directly from the patient. Most patients will feel gratified that their clinician gave thought to their situation. Further, by demonstrating reflection, the clinician models the importance of remaining curious about one's own thoughts and behaviors. Finally, follow-up questions and a well-formulated HPI tend to lead neatly to likely diagnoses and treatments.

Knowledge of what is expected in a write-up can help catalyze an effective interaction. On the other hand, knowing that a large amount of information will eventually be expected can lead interviewers to feel driven to get concrete information at the expense of other aspects of the interview. As described above, zealous pursuit of data is likely to lead to an inadequate interview.

Electronic medical records (EMRs) are a mixed blessing to the interviewer. Given the amount of time spent at a computer, it behooves the clinician to take advantage of the positive aspects of the EMR. What collateral history is available? What have previous clinicians seen in this patient? What have loved ones (or police officers) said about the patient? Does the patient seem different from before? What therapeutic intervention worked or failed? What lab results are available? Used in conjunction with the interview, the EMR can be invaluable.

The interview is incomplete without a written assessment, diagnosis, and plan. Compare these two summaries, written by psychiatrists who saw the same medically hospitalized patient:

## Conclusion #1

**Assessment/Diagnosis:** Alcohol use disorder, depressed.

**Plan:** AA.

## Conclusion #2

**Assessment:** Asked to evaluate a 50-year-old man for depression and alcohol abuse. He was seen to evaluate "depression" on day 3 of an unexpected hospitalization for acute, perforated appendicitis. He appears to have become depressed in the context of gradually escalating use of alcohol over the past 2 years. Functioning poorly at work and in his marriage. No suicidality, according to patient and wife. Aside from some tremor on hospital days 2–3, no withdrawal symptoms during this past week's hospitalization, though his currently heightened dysphoria might reflect withdrawal. Patient denies depression prior to 2 years ago, though he has strong family history of depression in multiple relatives. He claims that he shifted from drinking a few beers per week to a six pack every night just after his mother died, which was 2 years ago. Now drinks approximately 1–2 pints of vodka per day. MCV 100; AST/ALT: 85/40. Patient educated about several medication options (e.g., acamprosate, naltrexone, antidepressant medication, disulfiram) and treatment options (inpatient and outpatient rehabs, individual therapy) during the hospitalization. Patient strongly prefers to first try AA and then consider individual psychotherapy if his depression persists and/or he restarts drinking.

**Diagnosis:** Alcohol use disorder, moderate. Alcohol-induced depressive disorder.

**Plan:** AA.

The second conclusion is obviously more informative, but is it worth the time to summarize the situation when the diagnosis and treatment recommendation are the same? I would suggest that the longer assessment is indeed more useful. It may seem odd to emphasize the written report in a chapter on the interview, but, as with the development of the HPI, the interview itself is shaped by what is ultimately going to be expected. This is especially pertinent in regard to patients with co-occurring disorders. For example, it can be tempting to interview someone like the patient above and get stuck both with the diagnosis (e.g., Is the depression secondary to alcohol?) and with the ongoing treatment (He's refusing almost everything). In the face of uncertainty and likely nonadherence with an "optimal" treatment plan, the interviewer might decide to cut short both the interview and the write-up. If the clinician intends to write a well-thought-out HPI and concluding assessment, however, the interviewer's own thought is likely to become more reflective and sophisticated, the write-up will be more helpful to the next interviewer, and the interview itself stands a greater chance for success.

## KEY POINTS

- Nonverbal observation and conversation are crucial to effective evaluation.
- Without a working knowledge of psychiatry and substance abuse, the interviewer will get lost.
- Development of the history of the present illness guides the interview.
- The history of present illness is the creation of the interviewer.
- There is no single right way to interview.
- When in doubt, the interviewer should aim for warmth and curiosity.

# Questions

1. Which of the following is an example of the patient's chief complaint?

   A. "My parents are annoying."
   B. 36-year-old man with alcohol use disorder and a history of bipolar disorder.

C. Recurrent trials of antidepressants and mood stabilizers have failed.

D. Patient appears sullen, irritable, and with a mild intention tremor.

2. Which of the following components of a psychiatric interview focuses on a cross-sectional assessment of the patient?

A. History of present illness (HPI).

B. Mental status exam (MSE).

C. Assessment.

D. Treatment plan.

3. In the initial assesment of a patient for potentially co-occurring disorders, which one of the following is most crucial to clarify?

A. The single diagnosis that is causing the most difficulty.

B. All pertinent psychiatric diagnoses.

C. Sociopathy and illegal acts that might jeopardize treatment success.

D. The family's primary concerns.

# Reference

Mani N, Slevin N, Hudson A: What Three Wise Men have to say about diagnosis. BMJ 343:d7769, 2011 22187188

# Suggested Readings

Barnhill J: The psychiatric interview and mental status exam, in The American Psychiatric Publishing Textbook of Psychiatry, 6th Edition. Edited by Hales RE, Yudofsky SC, Roberts LW. Washington, DC, American Psychiatric Publishing, 2014, pp 3–30

MacKinnon RA, Michels R, Buckley PJ: The Psychiatric Interview in Clinical Practice, 3rd Edition. Arlington, VA, American Psychiatric Association Publishing, 2016

Miller WR, Rollnick S: Motivational Interviewing: Preparing People for Change, 3rd Edition. New York, Guilford, 2012

# 2

# THE COMPREHENSIVE ASSESSMENT

*Christine Yuodelis-Flores, M.D.*
*Richard K. Ries, M.D.*

A complete biopsychosocial assessment and integrated treatment plan can be crucial when working with patients who have co-occurring disorders (CODs). In this chapter, we describe a comprehensive evaluation that takes into account some of the unique aspects of this population. For example, in addition to evaluating the patient for relevant diagnoses and assessing their severity, the provider aims to determine the degree to which the mental illness is substance induced and understand how the mental and addictive disorders interact with each other and how the CODs affect psychosocial functioning.

This integrated evaluation will also assess the psychiatric symptoms, diagnoses, and treatment during past episodes of substance abuse and during periods of abstinence. This history will help clarify the role of the substance in maintaining or worsening the psychiatric symptoms and/ or affecting the psychiatric treatment.

The COD assessment is multidimensional and evaluates not only the degree of addiction and psychiatric illness but also withdrawal potential, biomedical complications, additional mental health conditions, readiness to change, relapse potential, and recovery environment. During the assessment process, the provider also investigates psychosocial issues such as current strengths, supports, limitations, and cultural barriers.

Finally, while conducting a COD assessment, the provider will assign the patient to one of the four categories in the Four Quadrant Model of Care for COD (Figure 2–1). This model is used to determine the appropriateness of the treatment setting based on severity of symptoms. The assessment for COD is integrated by examining the information concerning one disorder in light of evidence concerning the other disorder. As shown in Table 2–1, this 12-step process accords with Center for Substance Abuse Treatment (CSAT) Treatment Improvement Protocol 42 (Center for Substance Abuse Treatment 2005).

Use of this 12-step COD assessment process is illustrated in the following clinical case.

## Clinical Case

Douglas is a 45-year-old single male referred by his primary care provider for psychiatric evaluation and care. Douglas agreed to the evaluation because he has lost his job, is out of money, has no social supports, and has psychiatric symptoms and substance use that are increasingly problematic. His concerns can be divided into four categories: a preoccupation with mind control, mood and anxiety complaints, the use of psychoactive substances, and serious psychosocial stressors.

Douglas's most pressing and chronic concern relates to a sense that his mind is being controlled by people who are inserting thoughts, directing his behavior, and conducting experiments on him. He believes that 10 years ago a computer chip was somehow implanted in his head while he was sleeping. On awakening, he started to hear voices that comment on his actions or discuss what he will do next. At times the voices are overwhelming and prevent him from sleeping or concentrating at work. He feels agitated by these taunting voices. He believes that his friends and family were secretly involved with the insertion of the computer chip, so he cut contact with everyone he knew 5 years earlier.

He denies a family history of addictive disorders or mental illness. He had been taking antipsychotic and antidepressant medications for short periods in the past but stopped because

| I | | II | |
|---|---|---|---|
| Psychiatric disorder: **LOW** severity | Substance use disorder: **LOW** severity | Psychiatric disorder: **HIGH** severity | Substance use disorder: **LOW** severity |
| LOC: client served by primary care clinic | | LOC: client served by mental health center | |
| **III** | | **IV** | |
| Psychiatric disorder: **LOW** severity | Substance use disorder: **HIGH** severity | Psychiatric disorder: **HIGH** severity | Substance use disorder: **HIGH** severity |
| LOC: client served by addiction treatment program | | LOC: client served by mental health center with integrated COD program | |

FIGURE 2–1.    **Four-quadrant Model of Care for Co-occurring Disorders.**

COD=co-occurring disorder; LOC=locus of care.
*Source.* National Advisory Council, Substance Abuse and Mental Health Services Administration: *Improving Services for Individuals at Risk of, or With Co-occurring Substance-Related and Mental Health Disorders.* Rockville, MD, SAMHSA, 1997.

he felt that the medical providers believed it was "all in his head." He has consulted with several doctors, but their physical exams, X rays, and computed tomography scans found no chips in his head or neck. He has been unable to find a neurosurgeon willing to operate on him to remove the chip.

Douglas also reports anxiety and depressive symptoms. He describes chronic dysphoria, anhedonia, and a sense of hopelessness about whether his persecution will ever end. He has had thoughts of "ending it all" but has never planned or attempted suicide. He says he is always tired, partly because he sleeps so poorly. He says he often awakes after a few hours of sleep with a pounding heart rate, shortness of breath, sweats, a tremor, and voices screaming at him.

Douglas has a history of cannabis use since age 14 and currently smokes "two or three bowls" daily. He also drinks about six beers a night, most nights of the week. He denies any history of alcohol withdrawal symptoms or seizures, but he does note episodes of anxiety, sweating, tachycardia, and a tremor which he associates with the voices. While Douglas has no history of cocaine, gamma-hydroxybutyrate, hallucinogen, benzodiazepine,

---

**TABLE 2–1.** The 12-step assessment process for co-occurring
disorders (CODs)

---

1. Engage the client.

2. Upon receipt of appropriate client authorization(s), identify and contact collaterals (family, friends, other treatment providers) to gather additional information.

3. Screen and detect for COD.

4. Determine severity of mental and substance use disorders.

5. Determine appropriate care setting (e.g., inpatient, outpatient, residential).

6. Determine diagnosis (or diagnoses).

7. Determine disability and functional impairment.

8. Identify strengths and supports.

9. Identify cultural and linguistic needs and supports.

10. Identify additional problem areas to address (e.g., physical health, housing, vocational, educational, social, spiritual, cognitive).

11. Determine readiness for change.

12. Plan treatment.

---

*Source.*     Center for Substance Abuse Treatment 2005.

or opiate use/abuse, he did smoke and inject methamphetamine daily from age 24 to 35. After he developed psychotic symptoms, he gradually decreased his methamphetamine use and managed to completely stop on his own about 4 years ago. He has gradually increased his level of cannabis and alcohol use since stopping methamphetamine. He does not believe that the methamphetamine caused his auditory hallucinations because he stopped use so many years ago, and he believes that the cannabis and alcohol use have only helped his anxiety, dysphoria, and insomnia. He has never sought treatment for his substance use disorder (SUD).

Despite the severity of his symptoms, Douglas worked as a janitor and lived independently for the 5 years since rejecting his friends and family. He was, however, recently fired for absenteeism that he connects to increased substance use and worsening of his auditory hallucinations and feelings of persecution. He has just lost his unemployment benefits, is unable to pay his rent, and does not feel stable enough to seek employment.

Douglas was referred to the psychiatrist by a neurologist who had diagnosed hepatitis C during an evaluation for the mind-control chip. Douglas had generally refused medical and psychiatric care for many years, though he has sporadically agreed to take antidepressant and antipsychotic medication in the past. He agreed to see a psychiatrist at this time because he was feeling desperate.

At the end of the interview, Douglas is able to prioritize goals in treatment as 1) decrease or resolve the anxiety, depression, insomnia, and auditory hallucinations; 2) preserve his housing; 3) find a new job; and 4) seek treatment for his medical concerns.

# Discussion

In the 12-step process for evaluation of CODs (Table 2–1), the first step is to *engage the patient*. Eliciting the patient's perspective of his problem and desired treatment will help the provider to determine the degree of insight and willingness to accept treatment. The provider should be empathetic and offer hope and desire to work with the patient and treatment team to figure out the best plan of action.

Step 2 is to *identify collaterals and request signed releases of information in order to gather more information*. Although Douglas is isolated from friends and family, he has been treated by a variety of physicians. It will be important to identify those providers and review their assessments and treatment trials. A strong alliance may be able to overcome Douglas's possible reluctance to involve prior clinicians, especially if he recognizes that such information may allow a more effective plan of treatment.

Step 3, *screening and detecting for CODs*, can be tricky when patients have poor insight into illness. It is important to understand the chronology and course of his symptoms and the details of his substance use, though the approach needs to be tactful and may not be completed during the first visit. The assessment should include the severity of each substance use problem and mental illness. In Douglas's case, his methamphetamine use disorder was severe, but he appears to have attained long-term remission without formal treatment. He uses cannabis and alcohol daily, and they appear to be having a negative impact on his mental health. His psychosis appears to have been precipitated by his past methamphetamine use, but it may also be that the current psychosis was induced by or is associated with his cannabis and alcohol use.

Douglas has significant psychotic, depressive, and anxiety symptoms. It is possible that all of these symptoms are part of a primary psychosis such as schizophrenia or a substance-induced psychosis. He might also have some combination of a primary depressive disorder, a primary anxiety disorder, and/or a substance-induced depressive or anxiety disorder. The evaluation should also investigate possible mood swings or manic episodes, because Douglas would also be at risk for a diagnosis on the bipolar spectrum.

Step 4 is to *assess the severity of the disorders and determine the quadrant and locus of responsibility*. Douglas has many features that indicate a severe mental illness: a chronic and intense psychosis, a lack of insight, persistent dysphoria, insomnia, anxiety, and poor work and social functioning.

A suicide risk assessment is essential when evaluating a person with CODs. Does the patient wish he were dead or does he want to die? Does he have a plan for ending his life? How realistic is this plan and does he have the capability to execute the act? Has he ever tried to kill himself? What prevents him from killing himself?

The patient's potential to harm others should also be assessed. Does he feel a need to defend himself? Does he have a legal history, such as a history of assault or stalking behaviors? Given his psychosis, unintentional harm to others may result from misinterpretations of reality.

The severity of Douglas's SUDs is perhaps more moderate. He has maintained abstinence from methamphetamine and appears to have only mild withdrawal symptoms from alcohol and cannabis.

Using the Four Quadrants of Care for Co-occurring Disorders (Figure 2–1), the provider can assign Douglas to Quadrant II: more severe psychiatric illness and less severe SUD. When he was actively using daily intravenous methamphetamine, the SUD would be considered more severe.

Step 5 is to *determine the appropriate care setting*. Levels of care for CODs include

1. Treatment at the primary care level with consultation, intervention, and referral capabilities.
2. Outpatient addiction treatment program with psychiatric consultation and treatment.
3. Psychiatric outpatient program treatment with co-occurring addiction treatment.
4. Inpatient or residential addiction treatment with psychiatric consultation and treatment.
5. Medically managed intensive inpatient addiction treatment with psychiatric consultation and treatment.

6. Inpatient psychiatric hospitalization with medically managed addiction treatment.

When deciding on which level of care is needed for treatment of CODs, the provider must determine the severity of both disorders. In regard to addiction treatment, evaluation includes the patient's potential for overdose, withdrawal, and suicide. In addition to a severity assessment, it is important to take into consideration patient preference. In this case, Douglas has shown little desire for treatment of his substance use or psychiatric disorders. He has agreed to psychiatric assessment and to antipsychotic and antidepressant medications in the past. He would likely refuse inpatient psychiatric care but may accept the offer of outpatient psychiatric care and case management to help him with issues that bother him (e.g., insomnia, vocational and housing issues).

Regarding withdrawal potential, it will be important to ask the patient if he has had an extended time without alcohol or cannabis, how he tolerates days without substance use, and if he thinks he will have problems if he should suddenly stop use of alcohol or cannabis. Given the amount of substances consumed, his potential for serious withdrawal is low and can be managed on an outpatient basis. Since he is in Quadrant II, he will be most appropriately treated in a psychiatric outpatient COD program. Such a program tends to use a team approach consisting of psychiatrist, case manager, and addiction counselor. If his psychosis or depression becomes more severe or if he is actively suicidal or threatening to others, he would be more appropriate for psychiatric inpatient stabilization.

Step 6 is to *determine diagnoses*. In this case, Douglas has several diagnoses that will be more clearly determined over time and with collateral information. Enough information has been gathered to diagnose schizophrenia, but schizoaffective disorder and substance-induced psychosis are also possibilities. He also has a depressive disorder and an anxiety disorder, but it is unclear at this point whether they are primary or substance-induced.

Step 7 is to *determine disability and functional impairment*. Douglas has done remarkably well despite suffering from a severe mental illness. It is possible that his boss provided a low-stress work environment for him, but his functioning seems to have declined in the context of worsening cannabis and alcohol use. Douglas is more likely to enter into formal treatment if he is assured that vocational, housing, and medical services will be included in his treatment plan. The co-occurring treatment program is also likely to be more successful if he is able to develop relationships with mental health providers, addiction counselors, and other clients in the program. Additional support in the future can be developed through 12-step groups.

Step 8 is to *identify strengths and supports*. It is important to recognize that Douglas has strengths. He has a strong work ethic and had, until recently, successfully maintained employment despite chronic psychosis. He has never been psychiatrically hospitalized or attempted suicide. He successfully stopped using methamphetamines without addiction treatment. These indicate that he has reasonably intact impulse control. Although in this case, Douglas denies any social supports, this should be reevaluated as he gains trust and rapport with his treatment team. It is important to identify family members, treatment providers, friends, and organizations that the patient identifies as supportive in his or her life. If patients are socially isolated, the treatment team will often become their primary support.

Although the case does not focus on *identifying cultural needs and support* (Step 9), areas to explore include ethnicity, religious background and beliefs, gender identity and sexual orientation, learning disabilities, and educational level.

Step 10 is to *identify additional problem areas to address*.

*Medical issues* are potentially significant. Douglas's hepatitis C and history of intravenous methamphetamine use indicate a need to screen for additional diseases such as HIV disease, syphilis, and tuberculosis, as well as to investigate medical causes of psychosis and medical complications of his substance use. Screening labs should include urine toxicology as well as a comprehensive metabolic panel including liver function, renal function, electrolytes, blood sugar or hemoglobin $A_{1C}$, and thyroid function tests, as well as a complete blood count. Many co-occurring disorder programs are integrated and have medical providers associated with the program. After Douglas is engaged with his team, he should establish care with and be evaluated by a primary care provider. He should also be screened for dental problems, because severe tooth decay and gum disease are common in persons with methamphetamine dependence.

A *vocational evaluation* is a key element of a comprehensive COD program. Douglas is recently unemployed. Finding immediate employment might interfere with or even derail his psychiatric and addiction treatment, so the clinician should probably help him get short- or long-term disability. At the same time, Douglas wants to get a job, and so his recovery plan must include vocational and educational placement and support.

*Housing* is an important concern, since Douglas is unable to pay his rent. He would likely resist residential addiction and psychiatric care because he does not believe he requires addiction treatment. Community psychiatric treatment programs usually have housing specialists who may be able to help Douglas with housing options.

*Social and spiritual supports* can also be a crucial area of investigation. Douglas is estranged from family and friends. Peer support specialists, cognitive-behavioral therapy, recovery-oriented psychosocial group therapies, relapse prevention therapy, and educational classes will provide social supports for Douglas as he engages in treatment. Once he becomes engaged in treatment, 12-step groups and religious affiliations can also provide a more extensive sober support system.

*Step 11* is to *determine Douglas's readiness for change*. It is important to determine the stage of readiness for change for each substance use disorder. These stages include precontemplation, contemplation, preparation, action, and maintenance. In this case, Douglas is in the maintenance stage for his methamphetamine use disorder, but he is precontemplative regarding his alcohol and cannabis use.

Step 12 is to *plan treatment.* Treatment planning involves determining the stages of change for each identified problem, while remaining aware that different interventions will be necessary for different problems and stages of change. Creating a biopsychosocial treatment plan for each psychiatric and addiction diagnosis will help increase insight and willingness to enter into treatment. Treatment goals—both short- and long-term— should initially be derived primarily from the patient's perspective and then gradually altered and expanded as the assessment continues and the patient's insight and treatment progress.

## KEY POINTS

- Assessment of patients with co-occurring disorders involves a 12-step process. The process is multidimensional and includes an assessment of the mental illness and substance use disorder, their severities and complications, and how each disorder affects the other. It is also used to

  - determine the appropriate level of care and the patient's readiness for change, and to identify risks, strengths, and supports.

  - address medical, housing, vocational, cultural, social, spiritual, cognitive, and other concerns.

- Engaging the patient is essential for a comprehensive assessment and treatment plan and may take precedence over gathering information.

- Done correctly, this comprehensive biopsychosocial assessment will engage and motivate the patient, examine his or her perspectives and desires, identify problems, establish diagnoses, and lead to a comprehensive treatment plan.

# Questions

1. What is a core reason to use the Four Quadrant Model of Care for Co-occurring Disorders?

    A. It provides recommendations for psychiatric treatment alone.
    B. It helps clinicians select the appropriate level of care.
    C. It helps determine the stage of change of a patient.
    D. It helps guide medication management.

2. What is the value of determining a patient's readiness for change?

    A. It can replace a comprehensive psychiatric evaluation.
    B. It is essential in determining the types of interventions to implement.
    C. It can help the abstinent patient alone maintain abstinence.
    D. It is rarely valuable, as patients with SUDs seldom want to change.

3. The 12-step assessment process for co-occurring disorders

    A. Does not include a determination of readiness for change.
    B. Is multidimensional but does not take into account DSM-5.
    C. Is necessary to develop a comprehensive treatment plan.
    D. Includes establishing the diagnoses but not their severity.

# Reference

Center for Substance Abuse Treatment: Substance Abuse Treatment for Persons With Co-occurring Disorders. Treatment Improvement Protocol (TIP) Series 42 (DHHS Publ No SMA-05-3992). Rockville, MD, Substance Abuse and Mental Health Services Administration, 2005

# PART 2

## CO-OCCURRING DISORDERS

# DEPRESSIVE AND BIPOLAR DISORDERS

*Rocco A. Iannucci, M.D.*
*Roger D. Weiss, M.D.*

In order to effectively diagnose and treat the large number of people who have co-occurring depressive or bipolar disorders and substance use disorders (SUDs), the clinician must understand their interrelationships, pertinent demographic variables, and treatment strategies. In this chapter, we explore the connections between mood and substance use, with a focus on depression and cocaine.

A crucial statistical reality is that mood disorders are common, that substance use is common, and that the two are often found in the same person. There are many reasons for the common co-occurrence. Substance abuse can lead to serious depressive and manic symptoms via intoxication and withdrawal, for example, and chronic use of substances of abuse can lead to serious mood problems through a direct physiological effect or as a consequence of maladaptive behaviors and psychosocial stress. People may try to "self-medicate" depression by using sedating substances or stimulating substances, or both. Similarly, people with mania may try to reduce insomnia or agitation with sedating med-ications or try to trigger the pleasurable symptoms of hypomania with a stimulant. Other people with a mood disorder may just take whatever substance is available in order to change their mood symptoms (American Psychiatric Association 2013).

Not only do mood and substance use disorders commonly co-occur in the same individual, either diagnosis worsens the prognosis of the other. Each disorder is also associated with elevated risks of serious ad-verse outcomes such as accidental injury and suicide, with the greatest risk in persons with both classes of disorder. Although the body of re-search guiding best practices in the treatment of these co-occurring con-ditions is growing, many questions remain.

The third iteration of the National Epidemiologic Survey on Alcohol and Related Conditions (NESARC-III) provides a measure of prevalence and comorbidity rates for mood and substance use disorders. According to this survey, the 2012–13 lifetime prevalence of an alcohol use disorder in the United States was almost 30%; 13.9% of Americans had a lifetime history of severe alcohol use disorder, and 13.9% had exhibited any alcohol use disorder in the past year (Grant et al. 2015). The lifetime prevalence of a drug use disorder was nearly 10%, with 6.6% having a moderate-to-severe drug use disorder and nearly 4% meeting past-year criteria (Grant et al. 2004). Depressive and bipolar disorders are also common, with 9.3% meeting past-year criteria for any mood disorder (over 7% with past-year depression and 1.7% with mania in the past year) (Grant et al. 2016). Mood disorders are strongly associated with having a severe alcohol use disorder (odds ratio [OR]=1.8) or a moderate-to-severe drug use disorder (OR=2.2) in the past 12 months (Grant et al. 2004, 2015).

We present the case of a man with cocaine use and mood symptoms to illustrate common diagnostic challenges and to demonstrate a treatment approach for those with co-occurring depressive or bipolar disorders and SUDs.

---

## Clinical Case

Robert is 36-year-old attorney presenting at the urging of his husband, who unexpectedly came home during a weekday and discovered Robert smoking cocaine in their living room. Robert reports a 5-year history of cocaine use, beginning with casual use at a party with colleagues from his law office. He describes a pattern of use that was initially in his words "rec-reational," using intranasally every 1–2 weeks on Friday or Saturday nights. Shortly thereafter, he began to take an occasional "bump" at work, with the goal of enhancing energy and productivity. This pattern of use remained fairly stable for about 2 years, when he began to experience increasing stress and dissatisfaction at work, irritable and depressed mood, and increased frequency of cocaine use. In the past year, he used more days than not, generally in 2- to 3-day episodes of heavy use followed by abstinence for a few days to recover from the effects of cocaine. He has started to smoke "crack" cocaine and is now missing work on a frequent basis. Because of his husband's concern, Robert had recently been free of use for a period of 6 weeks, during which time he began attending Cocaine Anonymous.

While abstaining from cocaine, Robert experienced persistent low energy, poor concentration, depressed mood, and loss of interest and appetite over the course of 6 weeks, and he then resumed use. He reports past episodes of reckless behavior, irritable mood, and high energy interfering with sleep, largely in the context of escalating cocaine use. He also reports a history of depression in college, preceding any regular substance use. Known family history is significant for alcohol use disorder in his father, as well as depression or bipolar disorder in paternal aunts and uncles. Robert reports a desire to stop using cocaine because of problems at work and in his relationship. However, he worries about how to cope with low energy, depressed mood, and diminished sexual function that he experiences when not using cocaine. Robert reports surreptitious use of cocaine to enhance sexual experiences but denies sexual activity outside of the monogamous relationship with his husband.

# Discussion

This case illustrates some of the diagnostic challenges inherent to the co-occurrence of mood symptoms and SUDs. Individuals like Robert who use stimulants may induce symptoms that mimic bipolar disorder through a pattern of manic-like intoxication followed by withdrawal resembling depression. At the same time, individuals with SUDs are known to be at increased risk for both major depression and bipolar disorder. Robert shows further risk factors, including a family history of mood disorders, as well as a personal history of at least one major depressive episode preceding onset of cocaine use disorder. This information allows a diagnosis of major depressive disorder at the initial assessment but raises concern that the true diagnosis may be bipolar disorder. Robert also presents with symptoms consistent with a moderate-to-severe cocaine use disorder.

Clarifying the diagnostic question of an independent versus a substance-induced mood disorder in the presence of continuous drug or alcohol use is challenging. In this situation, it can be helpful to retrospectively review for historical symptoms during periods of abstinence, particularly periods lasting 30 days or longer. Substance-induced mood symptoms typically resolve over that time course. Likewise, careful family history can contribute to a full picture of the risk of an independent mood disorder. Nonetheless, it is important to note that many of those individuals initially diagnosed with substance-induced depression or mania will eventually be diagnosed as having an independent depressive or bipolar disorder (Tolliver and Anton 2015).

Patients presenting with histories of depressive or manic symptoms should undergo thoughtful, thorough examinations. Table 3–1 lists facets of the history that require particular attention in this population. Major depression, substance use disorders, and particularly bipolar disorders are all associated with significant elevation in suicide risk (Tolliver and Anton 2015). Continual assessment of suicide risk, starting at the initial assessment, is therefore essential.

History, physical examination, and laboratory testing facilitate assessment of medical factors contributing to mood symptoms. These may include thyroid illness, adrenal insufficiency, and other endocrine illnesses; hepatic, pulmonary, or renal disease; metabolic abnormalities; nutritional deficiencies; occult infections; and certain cancers. Sudden onset of behavior changes could reflect a neurological condition, such as dementia (especially the behavioral variant of frontotemporal dementia), multiple sclerosis, or stroke.

General screening tests are listed in Table 3–2, as are tests that may be pursued based on information gathered during the history and physical examination. Urine toxicology screening is generally advisable, because many persons with SUDs may be using multiple substances. Those who use stimulants will also commonly use sedatives such as alcohol, opioids, or benzodiazepines to moderate unpleasant sensations that occur as the initial euphoria begins to subside. Hence, cocaine use disorders co-occur with alcohol use disorder with a particularly high frequency. In addition, tobacco use disorder is very common among individuals with other SUDs and among those with mood disorders.

Collateral sources of information can be useful in the assessment of depressive and bipolar disorders and SUDs. Bipolar disorder manifests with both subjective symptoms and outward signs; the patient may have limited awareness of the latter, while familiar contacts can describe periods of

**TABLE 3–1.** Important elements elicited in assessment of patients with co-occurring substance-related and mood symptoms

| | |
|---|---|
| History of present illness | Elicit both current mood symptoms and substance-related symptoms. |
| Past psychiatric history | Focus on time periods prior to initiation of substance use and on any extended periods of abstinence (greater than 30 days). |
| | Review in detail suicidal ideation or suicide attempts and violent thoughts or behaviors. Include their relationship to mood symptoms and to substance use. |
| Medications | Gather a history of all medications, including nutritional supplements or complementary treatments. |
| | Review the history of medication adherence (overuse, taking by means other than prescribed, unilateral discontinuation). |
| Substance use history | Gather details of history, with attempt to clarify the presence or absence of mood symptoms. |
| | Clarify the relationship between mood symptoms and substance use, if any. |
| | Review what has been helpful or not helpful in the past, including attitudes to particular types of interventions, such as medications, psychotherapy, and self-help group involvement. |
| Family history | Review family history of substance use disorders, depressive and bipolar disorders, other psychiatric disorders, and suicide. |

rapid speech, increased impulsiveness, or other hallmark signs. At times, patients with SUDs may underrecognize or underreport problems related to their substance use. An involved partner, friend, or family member can add significantly to a thorough understanding of the scope of symptoms.

Substance use can cause medical illnesses and injuries, either as a direct result of substance use or connected to associated behaviors. In this case,

---

**TABLE 3–2.**  **Typical laboratory and diagnostic assessment of patients with mood and substance-related symptoms**

---

Complete blood count

Electrolytes

Blood urea nitrogen and creatinine

Thyroid-stimulating hormone

Transaminases, bilirubin, alkaline phosphatase, albumin, and total protein levels

Vitamin $B_{12}$ and folate levels

Viral hepatitis immunoassay

HIV immunoassay

Urine toxicology screen

Other tests (e.g., head CT or MRI, ECG, chest X ray, blood cultures) may be pursued based on particular symptoms

---

*Note.*   CT=computed tomography; ECG=electrocardiogram; MRI=magnetic resonance imaging.

Robert's use of cocaine may cause a potentially dangerous combination of vasoconstriction and acute hypertension that can predispose to cardiovascular complications such as angina pectoris, myocardial infarction, ventricular tachyarrhythmia, and hemorrhagic or nonhemorrhagic stroke. Intranasal use of cocaine causes vasoconstriction of the nasal mucosa, leading to symptoms of congestion, ulceration, or even perforation.

It is always important to take a thorough history of risky behaviors, including sexual practices. Manic patients can demonstrate hypersexual behavior. Likewise, substance use is often marked by impaired judgment and behavioral disinhibition. Stimulants in particular may be purposefully used to achieve disinhibition and to enhance sexual experiences and perceived performance. Over time, their use can lead to sexual dysfunction. Risk-taking may manifest as unsafe sexual or injection practices, leading to infection with HIV, hepatitis, endocarditis, or other diseases. Driving while intoxicated presents serious risk of accidental injury. Many individuals become disinhibited or even aggressive when intoxicated, increasing the likelihood of their becoming a victim or perpetrator of violence.

In Robert's case, although he denies risky sexual encounters outside a monogamous relationship, he acknowledges stimulant use during sexual behaviors. It will be important to address concerns he has about sexual health and to evaluate and treat any psychological or physiological conditions interfering with normal sexual function.

# Treatment

Helping a patient who is struggling with multiple serious illnesses calls on the clinician to set priorities while addressing each disorder. The most widespread approach in years past had generally been to help the patient establish a period of abstinence from substances before diagnosing and treating any mood symptoms. Mood disorders were treated, if at all, when it could be unambiguously established that they were independent and not substance-induced. This approach is called *sequential treatment.* Current practice recommendations involve the simultaneous, *integrated treatment* of depressive and bipolar disorders and SUDs, based on evidence that such an approach produces more favorable substance-related, and to some extent mood, outcomes (Morley et al. 2016; Weiss and Connery 2011).

One of the first decisions facing the clinician will be recommending the most appropriate setting and intensity of initial treatment. This evaluation should take into account potential for withdrawal, need for psychiatric stabilization to reduce risk of harm to self or others, and likelihood that a particular patient will respond to treatment in a given setting. While a full discussion of patient placement is beyond the scope of this chapter, the ASAM (American Society of Addiction Medicine) Criteria offer a systematic approach to forming such recommendations (Mee-Lee et al. 2013).

Notwithstanding the relatively small number of studies examining specific treatments in the subset of patients with co-occurring depressive and bipolar disorders and SUDs, there is a growing evidence base to guide best practice approaches to treatment. Motivational interviewing (MI), cognitive-behavioral therapy (CBT), contingency management (CM), and 12-step facilitation (TSF) can offer benefit to patients recovering from both classes of disorders. These approaches are reviewed briefly below.

## PSYCHOTHERAPEUTIC AND PSYCHOSOCIAL INTERVENTIONS

Motivational interviewing is an intervention that takes into account an individual's readiness to change substance-related behaviors, conceptualizing motivation as fluid and malleable under therapist influence. MI uses an explicitly client-centered, nonconfrontational approach to help bolster motivation to change. Based primarily on findings from studies involving patients with alcohol use disorders and depression, it appears to be a beneficial approach for those with co-occurring depression, yielding improved mood- and substance-related outcomes (DeVido and Weiss 2012), and can effectively be blended with CBT techniques (Riper et al. 2014).

Cognitive-behavioral approaches to SUDs generally combine a focus on internal and external cues related to substance use (including distorted thinking) with enhancement of skills to manage risky interpersonal situations and psychological factors. CBT has perhaps the strongest evidence base supporting use in treatment of SUDs and co-occurring depressive and bipolar disorders. Not only does CBT have positive effects in reducing substance use or mood when they occur as the sole diagnosis, it also has received significant study in those with co-occurring illnesses. Of note, CBT has been demonstrated to reduce depressive symptoms and substance use in people with co-occurring major depressive disorder and SUDs (Carroll 2004; Watkins et al. 2011). It also weakens the association between depressive symptoms and substance use, possibly by building alternative coping strategies when mood problems are experienced (Hunter et al. 2012).

A variant of CBT called *integrated group therapy* (IGT) has demonstrated particular efficacy in the treatment of patients with co-occurring bipolar disorder and SUDs. IGT is a 12-session group therapy that strongly emphasizes the interconnectedness between disorders, unifying them under the term "bipolar substance abuse." Important components of this approach include providing education about the similarities between maladaptive thoughts and behaviors underlying these disorders as well as about the bidirectional influence the illnesses exert on each other (Weiss and Connery 2011).

In three studies, IGT consistently produced better substance use outcomes even in comparison to a high-quality control intervention (i.e., group drug counseling). In one of these studies, IGT was also associated with a higher rate of achieving a "good clinical outcome," defined as abstinence from substances and no mood episode in the last month of treatment (Weiss et al. 2009). Note that IGT was conceived and tested as an "add-on" intervention, meant to complement typical treatment for bipolar disorder involving psychiatric management and mood stabilizers (Weiss and Connery 2011).

No discussion of psychosocial treatment for SUDs would be complete without mention of interventions that developed from the self-help (often called mutual-help) tradition, most prominently 12-step approaches. Twelve-step facilitation is a manualized, therapist-led intervention designed to introduce some 12-step principles and to encourage participants to engage in 12-step-based self-help groups. TSF is associated with improved substance and mood outcomes in depressed individuals with SUDs. However, after treatment completion, 12-step involvement and substance use outcomes may decline over time (Lydecker et al. 2010).

Contingency management, a behavioral approach grounded in principles of operant conditioning, has long been recognized as a robust treatment of stimulant use disorders. It has also shown benefit in a study of patients with stimulant use disorders and heterogeneous diagnoses of serious mental illness, many of whom had mood disorders (Carroll 2004; McDonell et al. 2013).

## PHARMACOLOGICAL INTERVENTIONS

As is the case for psychosocial treatments, more studies have investigated the use of medications to treat major depression than bipolar disorder co-occurring with SUDs. Although results have not always been consistent, research largely supports the use of antidepressants (including tricyclic agents and serotonin reuptake inhibitors, or SRIs) to treat depression in persons with SUDs, demonstrating a moderate effect on depressive symptoms and less effect on substance use outcomes (Nunes and Levin 2004; Pettinati et al. 2013). In practice, many clinicians favor use of SRIs because of these agents' generally more favorable safety profiles, despite some evidence that tricyclic antidepressants as a class may be more effective (Iovieno et al. 2011). As described below, SRIs may worsen outcomes for those with early-onset alcohol use disorder (Kranzler et al. 2011). There is less evidence to guide the psychopharmacological treatment of co-occurring bipolar disorder and SUDs. Valproic acid when added to lithium has shown promise for treatment of alcohol use disorder and bipolar disorder (Salloum et al. 2005). There is some limited evidence supporting potential benefit from citicoline or lamotrigine for treatment of co-occurring bipolar disorder and cocaine use disorder (Brown et al. 2012, 2015).

It should be noted that research on the treatment of co-occurring mood disorders and SUDs faces methodological challenges that may hinder discovery of effective interventions. First, the heterogeneity of the cohort under study can mask positive results in subpopulations of patients. For example, there is evidence that antidepressants are more effective for late-onset alcoholism, a finding that may be explained by polymorphisms of the gene encoding the serotonin transporter (Anthenelli et al. 2016). Moreover, for ethical reasons, many studies implement control procedures using a comparison group that is likely to effectively treat one or both disorders, making it more difficult to observe benefit for the studied intervention (Pettinati et al. 2013).

Notwithstanding, a reasonable approach is to treat both disorders while taking into account that it may be most appropriate to start medications sequentially rather than simultaneously. This will help prevent confusion about the cause of any potential adverse effects. Perhaps the strongest line of evidence for such an integrated pharmacotherapy approach is provided by studies of sertraline and naltrexone for co-occurring alcohol use disorder and major depression. The medication combination demonstrated improved drinking outcomes, as well as a trend toward significance in improved mood outcomes in comparison to placebo and to either agent alone (Pettinati et al. 2013).

The question of whether to treat depressive and bipolar disorders that are presumptively substance-induced remains unanswered. Arguments for treatment include studies demonstrating benefit from antidepressants in those with substance-induced depression, and even some demonstrated improvement in the absence of a mood disorder diagnosis (Pettinati et al. 2013). Furthermore, as described above, many people initially diagnosed with substance-induced disorders later have symptoms that meet criteria for an independent depressive or bipolar disorder (Morley et al. 2016). Substance-induced symptoms may be severe in nature and may involve elevated suicide risk. It is therefore often reasonable in these cases to initiate treatment likely to benefit both problems (such as CBT, possibly in combination with a medication targeting the SUD, such as naltrexone or acamprosate for alcohol use disorder when indicated). It is also reasonable to strongly consider starting an antidepressant (or mood stabilizer if appropriate) for more severe symptoms while diagnostic assessment is ongoing, with careful consideration of risks and benefits. These issues should be discussed thoroughly with the patient and should include education about substance-induced mood disorders, independent mood disorders, and the relative likelihood of each.

In Robert's case, the working diagnoses are cocaine use disorder and major depressive disorder, with the assumption that collateral information from supports yields no additional information to modify this assessment. Psychosocial interventions remain the mainstay of treatment for people with cocaine use disorder, because as of this writing there are no U.S. Food and Drug Administration (FDA)–approved medications for the treatment of cocaine use disorder. Contingency management, while backed by empirical evidence, is often difficult to access in clinical practice. CBT with a clinician experienced in treating both mood and SUDs would be an appropriate recommendation, as would 12-step or other mutual-help group involvement if the patient is amenable. An antidepressant would also be reasonable after educating Robert and his husband about risks such as precipitated suicidality or mania, how to identify these problems, and how to seek emergency treatment if they occur. The potential for sexual side effects should also be frankly discussed, along with other possible adverse effects. Should it become clear that Robert suffers from bipolar disorder, IGT in conjunction with psychopharmacological management (including mood stabilization) would be an appropriate course of action.

Tobacco use disorders often accompany other substance disorders. While a full discussion of treatment of nicotine use disorder is beyond the scope of this chapter, psychotherapeutic options (MI, CBT) and medications both have their places. Bupropion should be used with caution in patients with bipolar disorder because of risks associated with antidepressants. Varenicline, another effective medication for smoking cessation, carries an FDA-issued warning about neuropsychiatric symptoms and suicidality. These potential risks must be weighed against significant benefits of smoking cessation, keeping in mind that a large recent study showed no increase in adverse psychiatric events in those with mood disorders who were treated with either bupropion or varenicline (Anthenelli et al. 2016).

In addition to the limited but growing evidence base to guide treatments likely to benefit patients, some studies have raised questions about treatments that may carry additional risk for individuals with particular disorders. For instance, venlafaxine may impede improvements in cannabis use among heavy users by causing noradrenergic effects that mimic cannabis withdrawal (Kelly et al. 2014). Though commonly used to treat insomnia in those with alcohol use disorder, questions have been raised as to whether trazodone use is associated with a decreased likelihood of abstinence from alcohol (Friedmann et al. 2008), though others have not found this association (Kolla et al. 2011). Trazodone and other antidepressants could precipitate manic episodes or mood cycling in those with underlying bipolar disorder. This is not to imply that any of the treatments described above are absolutely contraindicated in the treatment of co-occurring mood and substance use disorders. Rather, risks and benefits must be thoroughly understood and carefully weighed by both physician and patient.

# Conclusion

The co-occurrence of mood and substance use disorders is a common and important clinical issue. While questions regarding best practice remain, there is a growing body of evidence to recommend integrated treatment of these disorders, including psychosocial and pharmacological approaches.

## KEY POINTS

- Mood and substance use disorders commonly co-occur. Clinicians should look carefully for substance use in patients with mood disorders and for mood problems in those with substance use disorders (SUDs).

- Among persons with SUDs, many of those who experience mood episodes will eventually have symptoms that meet criteria for an independent depressive or bipolar disorder.

- There is good evidence that co-occurring mood disorders and SUDs improve with treatment, including empirical information to recommend particular therapeutic approaches.

# Questions

1. Which medication combination has been shown to benefit patients with co-occurring major depressive disorder and alcohol use disorder?

    A. Sertraline and acamprosate.
    B. Desipramine and disulfiram.
    C. Venlafaxine and naltrexone.
    D. Sertraline and naltrexone.

2. Which psychotherapeutic approach has shown efficacy in three trials of treatment for co-occurring bipolar disorder and SUDs?

    A. Motivational interviewing (MI).
    B. Twelve-step facilitation.
    C. Group drug counseling.
    D. Integrated group therapy (IGT).

3. What psychosocial intervention both focuses on the connections among thoughts, feelings, and behaviors and has strong evidence for benefit in treating people with mood disorders, SUDs, or both?

    A. Cognitive-behavioral therapy (CBT).
    B. Twelve-step facilitation.
    C. Motivational interviewing.
    D. Alcoholics Anonymous.

# References

American Psychiatric Association: Diagnostic and Statistical Manual of Mental Disorders, 5th Edition. Arlington, VA, American Psychiatric Association, 2013

Anthenelli RM, Benowitz NL, West R, et al: Neuropsychiatric safety and efficacy of varenicline, bupropion, and nicotine patch in smokers with and without psychiatric disorders (EAGLES): a double-blind, randomised, placebo-controlled clinical trial. Lancet 387(10037):2507–2520, 2016 27116918

Brown ES, Sunderajan P, Hu LT, et al: A randomized, double-blind, placebo-controlled, trial of lamotrigine therapy in bipolar disorder, depressed or mixed phase and cocaine dependence. Neuropsychopharmacology 37(11):2347–2354, 2012 22669171

Brown ES, Todd JP, Hu LT, et al: A randomized, double-blind, placebo-controlled trial of citicoline for cocaine dependence in Bipolar I Disorder. Am J Psychiatry 172(10):1014–1021, 2015 25998279

Carroll KM: Behavioral therapies for co-occurring substance use and mood disorders. Biol Psychiatry 56(10):778–784, 2004 15556123

DeVido JJ, Weiss RD: Treatment of the depressed alcoholic patient. Curr Psychiatry Rep 14(6):610–618, 2012 22907336

Friedmann PD, Rose JS, Swift R, et al: Trazodone for sleep disturbance after alcohol detoxification: a double-blind, placebo-controlled trial. Alcohol Clin Exp Res 32(9):1652–1660, 2008 18616688

Grant BF, Stinson FS, Dawson DA, et al: Prevalence and co-occurrence of substance use disorders and independent mood and anxiety disorders: results from the National Epidemiologic Survey on Alcohol and Related Conditions. Arch Gen Psychiatry 61(8):807–816, 2004 15289279

Grant BF, Goldstein RB, Saha TD, et al: Epidemiology of DSM-5 Alcohol Use Disorder: results From the National Epidemiologic Survey on Alcohol and Related Conditions III. JAMA Psychiatry 72(8):757–766, 2015 26039070

Grant BF, Saha TD, Ruan WJ, et al: Epidemiology of DSM-5 Drug Use Disorder: Results from the National Epidemiologic Survey on Alcohol and Related Conditions–III. JAMA Psychiatry 73(1):39–47, 2016 26580136

Hunter SB, Witkiewitz K, Watkins KE, et al: The moderating effects of group cognitive-behavioral therapy for depression among substance users. Psychol Addict Behav 26(4):906–916, 2012 22564202

Iovieno N, Tedeschini E, Bentley KH, et al: Antidepressants for major depressive disorder and dysthymic disorder in patients with comorbid alcohol use disorders: a meta-analysis of placebo-controlled randomized trials. J Clin Psychiatry 72(8):1144–1151, 2011 21536001

Kelly MA, Pavlicova M, Glass A, et al: Do withdrawal-like symptoms mediate increased marijuana smoking in individuals treated with venlafaxine-XR? Drug Alcohol Depend 144:42–46, 2014 25283697

Kolla BP, Schneekloth TD, Biernacka JM, et al: Trazodone and alcohol relapse: a retrospective study following residential treatment. Am J Addict 20(6):525–529, 2011 21999497

Kranzler HR, Armeli S, Tennen H, et al: A double-blind, randomized trial of sertraline for alcohol dependence: moderation by age of onset [corrected] and 5-hydroxytryptamine transporter-linked promoter region genotype. J Clin Psychopharmacol 31(1):22–30, 2011 21192139

Lydecker KP, Tate SR, Cummins KM, et al: Clinical outcomes of an integrated treatment for depression and substance use disorders. Psychol Addict Behav 24(3):453–465, 2010 20853931

McDonell MG, Serbnik D, Angelo F, et al: Randomized controlled trial of contingency management for psycho-stimulant use in community mental health outpatients with co-occurring serious mental illness. Am J Psychiatry 170(1):94–101, 2013 23138961

Mee-Lee D, Shulman GD, Fishman MJ, et al: The ASAM Criteria: Treatment Criteria for Addictive, Substance-Related, and Co-Occurring Conditions. Carson City, NV, The Change Companies, 2013

Morley KC, Baillie A, Leung S, et al: Is specialized integrated treatment for comorbid anxiety, depression, and alcohol dependence better than treatment as usual in a public hospital setting? Alcohol Alcohol 51(4):402–409, 2016 26672793

Nunes EV, Levin FR: Treatment of depression in patients with alcohol or other drug dependence: a meta-analysis. JAMA 291(15):1887–1896, 2004 15100209

Pettinati HM, O'Brien CP, Dundon WD: Current status of co-occurring mood and substance use disorders: a new therapeutic target. Am J Psychiatry 170(1):23–30, 2013 23223834

Riper H, Andersson G, Hunter SB, et al: Treatment of comorbid alcohol use disorders and depression with cognitive-behavioural therapy and motivational interviewing: a meta-analysis. Addiction 109(3):394–406, 2014 24304463

Salloum IM, Cornelius JR, Daley DC, et al: Efficacy of valproate maintenance in patients with bipolar disorder and alcoholism: a double-blind placebo-controlled study. Arch Gen Psychiatry 62(1):37–45, 2005 15630071

Tolliver BK, Anton RF: Assessment and treatment of mood disorders in the context of substance abuse. Dialogues Clin Neurosci 17(2):181–190, 2015 26246792

Watkins KE, Hunter SB, Hepner KA, et al: An effectiveness trial of group cognitive behavioral therapy for patients with persistent depressive symptoms in substance abuse treatment. Arch Gen Psychiatry 68(6):577–584, 2011 21646576

Weiss RD, Connery HS: Integrated Group Therapy for Bipolar Disorder and Substance Abuse. New York, Guilford, 2011

Weiss RD, Griffin ML, Jaffee WB, et al: A "community-friendly" version of integrated group therapy for patients with bipolar disorder and substance dependence: a randomized controlled trial. Drug Alcohol Depend 104(3):212–219, 2009 19573999

# 4

# ANXIETY DISORDERS

*Rebecca A. Nejat, M.D.*
*Maria Andrea Baez, M.D.*

Anxiety and psychoactive substance use often co-occur. Substances like cocaine and marijuana can directly and acutely induce anxiety. They can also contribute to the development of chronic anxiety, in which symptoms can become significant in the presence or absence of recent, persistent substance use. Sedating substances like benzodiazepines and alcohol are often used to reduce anxiety, though chronic use may be associated with enhanced anxiety, and even mild withdrawal from these sedating substances typically leads to anxiety. In one study, almost half of people with a lifetime diagnosis of generalized anxiety disorder (GAD) also had a lifetime diagnosis of a substance use disorder (SUD), while almost 20% of people with any SUD have an anxiety disorder that predated their debilitating substance use (Alegría et al. 2010; Grant et al. 2004). In other words, these co-occurring disorders (CODs) are very common, particularly in treatment settings.

This chapter focuses on diagnostic and therapeutic interventions for this particular patient population. For example, we describe how to identify the primary diagnosis and discuss why this is therapeutically important. We also discuss the abuse of prescribed sedating medications, iatrogenic difficulties, and the importance of focusing on both the anxiety disorder and the SUD from the very onset of the evaluation and treatment.

In the following case we describe a middle-age man whose anxiety worsened in the setting of benzodiazepine and alcohol use. Although CODs that involve anxiety and substances can be complicated, this case touches on the core principles that can be applied to virtually any patient with both anxiety and substance use disorders.

## Clinical Case

Henry is a 53-year-old domiciled, married, and self-employed man with no formal past medical history who has never seen a psychiatrist. He was brought into the psychiatric emergency room by his wife after telling her he was so overwhelmed by insomnia and constant "sky-high" anxiety that he needed help.

The patient states that he has always been a "worrier." He states that he has had long-standing concerns about his overall state of health (although he sees doctors regularly and has no chronic medical conditions) and about his financial future. However, although he has always been a "worrier," these fears have never stopped him from being productive, enjoying his life, or having meaningful relationships with others. He immigrated to the United States at age 21, pursued a graduate degree in engineering, and is self-employed in real estate development.

He reports 2 years of financial stress. Since that time, he has been consumed with constant excessive worry about his health, about his wife's health, about their finances, and about accomplishing his daily tasks. He feels restless constantly and feels that the restlessness and constant anxiety make him unable to focus at work, which worsens his anxiety further. He states he is unable to stop himself from constantly focusing on these fears and is not relieved when others reassure him. He states that worst of all, despite being extremely fatigued at the end of the day, he is unable to fall asleep due to anxious ruminations. He states it takes him about 3–4 hours to fall asleep and then he wakes up after just 6 hours of sleep.

Approximately 12 months ago the patient saw his primary care doctor for insomnia. His doctor prescribed alprazolam, initially at 0.5 mg QHS, but because of continued anxiety, the dose was slowly increased and the patient is now taking more than recommended by his doctor. He is currently taking 4 mg of alprazolam at bedtime as well as 1–2 mg as needed during the day.

Henry also admits that, while he has not told his primary care doctor, he has found over time that increasing the amount he drinks with dinner helps him fall asleep. He states he has been drinking three shots of vodka at night as well as having 1–2 beers during the day for the past 6 months. He states that while this regimen helps him fall asleep, he awakens every night around 3 A.M. with intensely high anxiety and palpitations, which prevent him from falling back asleep. He states he feels guilty about his drinking but has been unable to cut down because of cravings, desire to immediately relieve anxiety, and insomnia. While the patient denies spontaneous suicide thoughts and denies active plans to end his life, he states that he would not want to live if told his anxiety would never go away. He denies anhedonia, use of other substances, hallucinations, or violent thoughts. He begs multiple times, "Doctor please, just give me something for sleep, something stronger than Xanax."

# Discussion

Henry's case highlights the interrelations between anxiety and substance use. As mentioned earlier, it can be challenging to identify which came first, the anxiety disorder or the SUD. Further, other factors (e.g., genetics, trauma) may lead to anxiety disorders and SUDs developing seemingly independently of each other as well.

The single most useful tool for diagnostic clarity is creating a timeline of symptoms and behaviors. It is particularly useful to identify the presence or absence of anxiety during periods of abstinence. Substance-induced anxiety symptoms will improve in the absence of substance use. It is also important to clarify whether anxiety symptoms were significant prior to the onset of clinically relevant substance use. Although relatively nonspecific, a family history of anxiety disorders is often found in people with a primary anxiety disorder (Hartwell et al. 2014) (see interview tips in Table 4–1).

On the basis of a targeted interview, we can begin to form a differential diagnosis for a patient who presents with symptoms of anxiety (Table 4–2). In Henry's case, we notice that he had symptoms of GAD for at least 1 year prior to starting regular use of benzodiazepines or alcohol. These symptoms occurred during a time of abstinence. We can therefore diagnose him with an independent anxiety disorder, GAD.

His need for immediate relief from anxiety prompted him to start using large amounts of benzodiazepines, which resulted in a benzodiazepine (or sedative-hypnotic) use disorder. Additionally, the patient has had

---

**TABLE 4–1. Interview inquiries to help differentiate primary anxiety disorder from substance-induced anxiety disorder**

---

Ask when the longest period of abstinence has been; assess whether patient had anxiety symptoms during that time.

Ask whether the patient had onset of anxiety symptoms prior to starting to abuse substance.

Inquire about family history of a primary anxiety disorder.

Determine age at onset of anxiety symptoms.

Screen all patients who arrive with chief complaint of anxiety for substance use disorder, and vice versa.

---

a pattern of excessive and problematic alcohol use for the past 6 months and thus also has an alcohol use disorder. Henry's consistent use of alcohol and sedative-hypnotics likely cause intermittent periods of withdrawal, which wake him from sleep with anxiety and palpitations. This cycle is known as the "forward feeding cycle" of alcohol and anxiety symptoms (Kushner et al. 2000).

Alcohol is particularly correlated with anxiety (Alegría et al. 2010; Grant et al. 2005; Smith and Book 2010). In one study, of patients whose alcohol use met criteria for alcohol use disorder, 46% also had symptoms that met criteria for GAD (Smith and Book 2010).

Drugs of abuse can be divided into three groups with regard to anxiety: those that relieve anxiety with intoxication and precipitate anxiety with withdrawal (e.g., alcohol); those that exacerbate anxiety in intoxication (e.g., cocaine); and those such as marijuana and nicotine that may heighten or reduce anxiety (Table 4–3) (Green et al. 2003; Hartwell et al. 2014; Morissette et al. 2007; Raphael et al. 2005).

# Treatment

Henry has a primary anxiety disorder, and it is clear that he is using alcohol and benzodiazepines to self-medicate. As discussed above, other patients develop an anxiety disorder in the context of a SUD, and anxiety disorders and SUDs may also seem to develop independently. Regardless, all too often, clinicians choose to focus on one half of the patient's problems, leading to undertreatment and prolonged periods of distress and dysfunction. Once multiple disorders have developed, they all need to be addressed.

---

**TABLE 4–2. Differential diagnosis of anxiety symptoms**

Primary anxiety disorder
    Social anxiety disorder
    Panic disorder
    Agoraphobia
    Generalized anxiety disorder
    Unspecified anxiety disorder
Substance-induced anxiety disorder (in intoxication or withdrawal)
Medication-induced anxiety disorder
Anxiety disorder due to another medical condition
Posttraumatic stress disorder

---

As is true for other co-occurring psychiatric conditions, treatment is most effective when it combines psychosocial, psychotherapeutic, and pharmacological interventions. General treatment considerations are reviewed in Table 4–4.

## PSYCHOTHERAPEUTIC AND PSYCHOSOCIAL INTERVENTIONS

Psychotherapeutic treatments for both anxiety disorders and SUDs tend to focus on anxiety tolerance, skill building, and coping techniques. Cognitive-behavioral therapy (CBT) appears especially effective for both disorders (Hartwell et al. 2014; McHugh et al. 2010; Otte 2011). Patients with social anxiety disorder may not be able to tolerate group-based treatments; instead, they may require either individual therapy or treatment of the social anxiety disorder before a group treatment and/ or a 12-step program are initiated (Book et al. 2009; Hartwell et al. 2014).

## PHARMACOLOGICAL INTERVENTIONS

The gold standard for pharmacological treatment is treatment of each individually diagnosed disorder (Ravindran and Stein 2010). A core additional principle is to prescribe the least habit-forming pharmacological agent for the anxiety, particularly avoiding harmful interactions between the substance of abuse and the prescribed medication (Hartwell et al. 2014). Benzodiazepines are frequently prescribed for anxiety in the non-SUD population, but they are not recommended for treatment of anxiety in patients with an active SUD because of their abuse potential.

TABLE 4–3.  Effects of substances of abuse on anxiety symptoms

| Drug | Effect on anxiety symptoms |
| --- | :---: |
| Alcohol | |
| Intoxication | ↓ |
| Withdrawal/chronic use | ↑ |
| Nicotine | |
| Intoxication | ? |
| Withdrawal/chronic use | ↑ |
| Opiates | |
| Intoxication | ↓ |
| Withdrawal/chronic use | ↑ |
| Marijuana | |
| Intoxication | ? |
| Withdrawal/chronic use | ↑ |
| Stimulants | |
| Intoxication | ↑ |
| Chronic use | ↑ |

One exception to this rule may be the careful and monitored use of benzodiazepines to imminently lower acute panic in panic disorder.

The first-choice medications for treatment of most anxiety disorders are selective serotonin reuptake inhibitors (SSRIs), which are generally considered safe and efficacious in the individual with CODs (Ravindran and Stein 2010). Serotonin-norepinephrine reuptake inhibitors (SNRIs) have a similar safety and efficacy profile (Ravindran and Stein 2010). There is some specific evidence that supports the use of mirtazapine in panic disorder and social anxiety disorder (Sarchiapone et al. 2003; Van Veen et al. 2002). Second- and third-line drugs for GAD include imipramine, buspirone, pregabalin, bupropion XL, trazodone, mirtazapine, hydroxyzine, olanzapine, and risperidone (Canadian Psychiatric Association 2006; Hartwell et al. 2014). However, in the dually diagnosed patient, bupropion is generally avoided because of increased seizure risk (particularly with alcohol and benzodiazepine use), and it may exacerbate anxiety in some patients. Tricyclic antidepressants and monoamine oxidase inhibitors are often reserved for treatment of refractory cases (Ravindran and Stein 2010). Gabapentin has demonstrated some efficacy in treatment of social anxiety disorder (Pande et al. 1999).

TABLE 4–4. Guidelines for treating co-occurring primary anxiety
disorder and substance use disorder

Focus on timeline of symptoms during the interview for diagnostic
clarity.

Consider combining psychosocial therapies and pharmacological
agent treatment for most patients with co-occurring substance use
disorder and anxiety disorder.

Consider groups (e.g., 12-step programs) or group-based treatments
for patients with primary anxiety disorders, except for patients
with social anxiety disorder (for whom group therapy may be
contraindicated).

If co-occurring primary anxiety and substance diagnoses exist,
prescribe medications for both the anxiety disorder and for the
specific substance use disorder.

Medications such as naltrexone for alcohol use disorder or buprenorphine for opioid use disorder can generally be safely used to treat SUDs
in patients who are also being treated pharmacologically for their anxiety (Hartwell et al. 2014). Gabapentin is unique in that there is evidence
for its effectiveness in treating both anxiety (as discussed above) and
SUDs, including marijuana use disorder and alcohol use disorder (Furieri and Nakamura-Palacios 2007; Sherman and McRae-Clark 2016). In
the case of Henry, for example, he might be started on naltrexone and an
SSRI while taking advantage of such interventions as motivational interviewing, CBT to enhance coping skills, and a 12-step program.

# Conclusion

Anxiety and substance use often co-occur. The clinician plays a vital role
in elucidating whether anxiety occurs independent of substance use
(and thus is part of a primary anxiety disorder) or whether the anxiety is
secondary to substance use (i.e., a substance-induced anxiety disorder).
Focusing on whether anxiety exists during periods of abstinence is critical to establishing a diagnosis. When primary anxiety disorders and
SUDs co-occur, treating both simultaneously with psychosocial, psychotherapeutic, and pharmacological interventions is recommended.

## KEY POINTS

- Patients with anxiety may have a primary anxiety disorder, a substance use disorder (SUD), a substance-induced anxiety disorder, or a combination of these diagnoses.
- Alcohol use disorder is a common comorbidity with primary anxiety disorders.
- Choosing therapies (both behaviorally based and medication based) that target both anxiety and substance use, when these disorders co-occur, is important in effective treatment.
- Group-based therapies are generally contraindicated in patients with social anxiety disorder.
- There are some unique considerations involved in the pharmacological treatment of concurrent anxiety and SUD, including avoiding habit-forming medications when possible (e.g., benzodiazepines) and avoiding bupropion if there is a concern for lowering the seizure threshold (e.g., in alcohol and benzodiazepine use disorders).

# Questions

1. The best way to differentiate substance-induced anxiety disorder from a primary anxiety disorder is based on

    A. Duration of anxiety symptoms.
    B. Relationship of anxiety symptoms to periods of use or abstinence.
    C. Responsiveness to medications.
    D. Family history of anxiety disorder.

2. Ms. G is a 42-year-old female who comes to your office with complaints of excessive alcohol use hindering her ability to maintain her job and stable interpersonal relationships as well as impairing social anxiety. You determine, based on the timeline of her symptoms, that her symptoms meet diagnostic criteria for social anxiety disorder and alcohol use disorder. She has never taken psychiatric medications before. Optimal initial treatment would include

    A. Disulfram and a selective serotonin reuptake inhibitor (SSRI).
    B. Trial of clonazepam and SSRI.

    C. Trial of an SSRI, naltrexone, and individual cognitive-behavioral therapy (CBT).

    D. Trial of SSRI, naltrexone, and a 12-step-based group abstinence program.

3. Which of the following medications should generally be avoided in a patient with both a primary anxiety disorder and an alcohol use disorder?

    A. Clonidine.

    B. Naltrexone.

    C. Lorazepam.

    D. Acamprosate.

# References

Alegría AA, Hasin DS, Nunes EV, et al: Comorbidity of generalized anxiety disorder and substance use disorders: results from the National Epidemiologic Survey on Alcohol and Related Conditions. J Clin Psychiatry 71(9):1187–1195, quiz 1252–1253, 2010 20923623

Book SW, Thomas SE, Dempsey JP, et al: Social anxiety impacts willingness to participate in addiction treatment. Addict Behav 34(5):474–476, 2009 19195794

Canadian Psychiatric Association: Clinical practice guidelines. Management of anxiety disorders. Can J Psychiatry 51(8)(Suppl 2):9S–91S, 2006 16933543

Furieri FA, Nakamura-Palacios EM: Gabapentin reduces alcohol consumption and craving: a randomized, double-blind, placebo-controlled trial. J Clin Psychiatry 68(11):1691–1700, 2007 18052562

Grant BF, Stinson FS, Dawson DA, et al: Prevalence and co-occurrence of substance use disorders and independent mood and anxiety disorders: results from the National Epidemiologic Survey on Alcohol and Related Conditions. Arch Gen Psychiatry 61(8):807–816, 2004 15289279

Grant BF, Hasin DS, Blanco C, et al: The epidemiology of social anxiety disorder in the United States: results from the National Epidemiologic Survey on Alcohol and Related Conditions. J Clin Psychiatry 66(11):1351–1361, 2005 16420070

Green B, Kavanagh D, Young R: Being stoned: a review of self-reported cannabis effects. Drug Alcohol Rev 22(4):453–460, 2003 14660135

Hartwell KJ, Magro TK, Brady KT: Co-occurring addiction and anxiety disorders, in The ASAM Principles of Addiction Medicine, 5th Edition. Edited by Ries RK, Fiellin DA, Miller SC, et al: Philadelphia, PA, Lippincott Williams & Wilkins, 2014, pp 1333–1345

Kushner MG, Abrams K, Borchardt C: The relationship between anxiety disorders and alcohol use disorders: a review of major perspectives and findings. Clin Psychol Rev 20(2):149–171, 2000 10721495

McHugh RK, Hearon BA, Otto MW: Cognitive behavioral therapy for substance use disorders. Psychiatr Clin North Am 33(3):511–525, 2010 20599130

Morissette SB, Tull MT, Gulliver SB, et al: Anxiety, anxiety disorders, tobacco use, and nicotine: a critical review of interrelationships. Psychol Bull 133(2):245–272, 2007 17338599

Otte C: Cognitive behavioral therapy in anxiety disorders: current state of the evidence. Dialogues Clin Neurosci 13(4):413–421, 2011 22275847

Pande AC, Davidson JR, Jefferson JW, et al: Treatment of social phobia with gabapentin: a placebo-controlled study. J Clin Psychopharmacol 19(4):341–348, 1999 10440462

Raphael B, Wooding S, Stevens G, Connor J: Comorbidity: cannabis and complexity. J Psychiatr Pract 11(3):161–176, 2005 15920390

Ravindran LN, Stein MB: The pharmacologic treatment of anxiety disorders: a review of progress. J Clin Psychiatry 71(7):839–854, 2010 20667290

Sarchiapone M, Amore M, De Risio S, et al: Mirtazapine in the treatment of panic disorder: an open-label trial. Int Clin Psychopharmacol 18(1):35–38, 2003 12490773

Sherman BJ, McRae-Clark AL: Treatment of cannabis use disorder: current science and future outlook. Pharmacotherapy 36(5):511–535, 2016 27027272

Smith JP, Book SW: Comorbidity of generalized anxiety disorder and alcohol use disorders among individuals seeking outpatient substance abuse treatment. Addict Behav 35(1):42–45, 2010 19733441

Van Veen JF, Van Vliet IM, Westenberg HG: Mirtazapine in social anxiety disorder: a pilot study. Int Clin Psychopharmacol 17(6):315–317, 2002 12409686

# POSTTRAUMATIC STRESS DISORDER

*J. David Stiffler, M.D.*
*Grace Hennessy, M.D.*

A significant portion of the general population will experience trauma in their lifetime (Kessler et al. 1995). Some will go on to develop posttraumatic stress disorder (PTSD), which, by definition, involves four clusters of symptoms (American Psychiatric Association 2013) (Table 5–1, B–E). Individuals with PTSD are at increased risk of having a substance use disorder (SUD), and having a SUD puts one at risk for developing PTSD (Saladin et al. 2014). It can be challenging to treat individuals diagnosed with both PTSD and SUDs because symptoms of both disorders can overlap (Table 5–2), leading to difficulties in making an accurate diagnosis. Furthermore, the presence of these commonly co-occurring disorders (Table 5–3) worsens the overall prognosis for each of them (Schäfer and Navajits 2007).

The following clinical case involves a young Marine who develops PTSD and multiple SUDs during and after his service in Afghanistan.

**TABLE 5–1. DSM-5 diagnostic criteria for posttraumatic stress disorder**

A. Exposure to actual or threatened death, serious injury, or sexual violence in one (or more) of the following ways:

1. Directly experiencing the traumatic event(s).
2. Witnessing, in person, the event(s) as it occurred to others.
3. Learning that the traumatic event(s) occurred to a close family member or close friend. In cases of actual or threatened death of a family member or friend, the event(s) must have been violent or accidental.
4. Experiencing repeated or extreme exposure to aversive details of the traumatic event(s).

B. Presence of one (or more) of the following intrusion symptoms associated with the traumatic event(s), beginning after the traumatic event(s) occurred:

1. Recurrent, involuntary, and intrusive distressing memories of the traumatic event(s).
2. Recurrent distressing dreams in which the content and/or affect of the dream are related to the traumatic event(s).
3. Dissociative reactions (e.g., flashbacks) in which the individual feels or acts as if the traumatic event(s) were recurring.
4. Intense or prolonged psychological distress at exposure to internal or external cues that symbolize or resemble an aspect of the traumatic event(s).
5. Marked physiological reactions to internal or external cues that symbolize or resemble an aspect of the traumatic event(s).

C. Persistent avoidance of stimuli associated with traumatic event(s), beginning after the traumatic event(s) occurred, as evidenced by one or both of the following:

1. Avoidance of or efforts to avoid distressing memories, thoughts, or feelings about or closely associated with the traumatic event(s).
2. Avoidance of or efforts to avoid external reminders (people, places, conversations, activities, objects, situations) that arouse distressing memories, thoughts, or feelings about or closely associated with the traumatic event(s).

**TABLE 5–1.** DSM-5 diagnostic criteria for posttraumatic stress disorder (*continued*)

D. Negative alterations in cognitions and mood associated with the traumatic events(s), beginning or worsening after the traumatic event(s) occurred, as evidenced by two (or more) of the following:

1. Inability to remember an important aspect of the traumatic event(s).
2. Persistent and exaggerated negative beliefs or expectations about oneself, others, or the world.
3. Persistent, distorted cognitions about the cause or consequences of the traumatic event(s) that lead the individual to blame himself/herself or others.
4. Persistent negative emotional state.
5. Markedly diminished interest or participation in significant activities.
6. Feelings of detachment or estrangement from others.
7. Persistent inability to experience positive emotions.

E. Marked alterations in arousal and reactivity associated with traumatic event(s), beginning or worsening after the traumatic event(s) occurred, as evidenced by two (or more) of the following:

1. Irritable behavior and angry outbursts (with little or no provocation) typically expressed as verbal or physical aggression toward people or objects.
2. Reckless or self-destructive behavior.
3. Hypervigilance.
4. Exaggerated startle response.
5. Problems with concentration.
6. Sleep disturbance.

F. Duration of the disturbance (Criteria B, C, D, and E) is more than 1 month.

G. The disturbance causes clinically significant distress or impairment in social, occupational, or other important areas of functioning.

H. The disturbance is not attributable to the physiological effects of a substance or another medical condition.

*Source.* Adapted from American Psychiatric Association: *Diagnostic and Statistical Manual of Mental Disorders,* 5th Edition. Arlington, VA, American Psychiatric Association, 2013. Copyright © 2013 American Psychiatric Association. Used with permission.

**TABLE 5–2.** Overlap of DSM-5 symptoms of intoxication and withdrawal with posttraumatic stress disorder (PTSD) symptoms

| Substance | Intoxication or withdrawal | Effect | Overlap with PTSD symptoms |
|---|---|---|---|
| Alcohol | Withdrawal | Autonomic hyperactivity (sweating, tachycardia) | Marked physiological reactions to cues that resemble the traumatic event |
|  |  | Psychomotor agitation | Alterations in arousal and reactivity |
|  |  | Anxiety | Sleep disturbances |
|  |  | Insomnia |  |
| Caffeine | Intoxication | Restlessness | Alterations in arousal and reactivity |
|  |  | Nervousness | Hypervigilance, exaggerated startle response |
|  |  | Psychomotor agitation | Irritable behavior, angry outbursts |
|  |  | Insomnia | Sleep disturbances |
|  |  | Tachycardia | Marked physiological reactions to cues that resemble the traumatic event |
| Caffeine | Withdrawal | Dysphoric/depressed mood | Persistent negative emotional state |
|  |  | Irritability | Alterations in arousal and reactivity |
|  |  | Difficulty concentrating | Irritable behavior |
|  |  |  | Problems with concentration |

**TABLE 5–2.** Overlap of DSM-5 symptoms of intoxication and withdrawal with posttraumatic stress disorder (PTSD) symptoms *(continued)*

| Substance | Intoxication or withdrawal | Effect | Overlap with PTSD symptoms |
|---|---|---|---|
| Cannabis | Intoxication | Anxiety | Alterations in arousal and reactivity |
| | | Tachycardia | Marked physiological reactions to cues that resemble the traumatic event |
| Hallucinogen | Intoxication | Psychological or behavioral changes | Alterations in arousal and reactivity |
| | | | Irritable behavior, angry outbursts |
| | | Tachycardia | Marked physiological reactions to cues that resemble the traumatic event |
| | | Sweating, palpitations | |
| Phencyclidine | Intoxication | Behavioral changes—psycho-motor agitation, assaultiveness | Marked alterations in arousal and reactivity |
| | | | Irritable behavior, angry outbursts |
| | | Tachycardia | Marked physiological reactions to cues that resemble the traumatic event |
| Opioid | Withdrawal | Dysphoric mood | Persistent negative emotional state |
| | | Insomnia | Sleep disturbances |

**TABLE 5–2.** Overlap of DSM-5 symptoms of intoxication and withdrawal with posttraumatic stress disorder (PTSD) symptoms (*continued*)

| Substance | Intoxication or withdrawal | Effect | Overlap with PTSD symptoms |
|---|---|---|---|
| Sedative, hypnotic, anxiolytic | Withdrawal | Autonomic hyperactivity<br>Psychomotor agitation<br>Anxiety<br>Insomnia | Marked physiological reactions to cues that resemble the traumatic event<br>Marked alterations in arousal and reactivity<br>Sleep disturbances |
| Stimulant | Intoxication | Tachycardia<br>Perspiration<br>Psychomotor agitation | Marked physiological reactions to cues that resemble the traumatic event<br>Marked alterations in arousal and reactivity |
| Tobacco | Withdrawal | Anxiety<br>Restlessness<br>Irritability<br>Frustration, anger<br>Difficulty concentrating<br>Depressed mood<br>Insomnia | Marked alterations in arousal and reactivity<br>Irritable behavior, angry outbursts<br>Problems with concentration<br>Persistent negative emotional state<br>Sleep disturbances |

**TABLE 5–3.** Prevalence of comorbid diagnoses of posttraumatic stress disorder (PTSD) and substance use disorders (SUDs)

| Primary disorder | Comorbid diagnosis | Prevalence | Reference |
|---|---|---|---|
| PTSD | Any SUD—lifetime | 22%–43% | Jacobsen et al. 2001 |
| | Alcohol use disorder—current | 36%–52% | Reynolds et al. 2005 |
| | Tobacco use disorder—current | 34%–86% | Fu et al. 2007 |
| | Other substance use disorders—current | 36%–52% | Trafton et al. 2006 |
| SUDs | PTSD—lifetime | 30%–58% | Reynolds et al. 2005 |
| | PTSD—current | 20%–38% | Reynolds et al. 2005 |

The case presentation and discussion will highlight diagnostic difficulties and ways to organize potentially complex clinical presentations. Central to the initial assessment is the importance of identifying PTSD, but it is also important to consider SUDs that might be minimized by the patient. In the treatment section, we present the evidence for various treatment models and highlight some concrete therapeutic strategies that have been found to be effective when working with this particular patient population.

## Clinical Case

Joe is a 25-year-old man who lives with his wife and two young children. The middle of three children, Joe and his siblings were raised by his mother, who struggled to keep a job, battled depression, and was addicted to heroin. Joe's father was physically abusive, had problems with alcohol and crack, and was often absent from the family for several months at a time. Despite these adversities, Joe graduated high school and married his high school sweetheart, who gave birth to their son when Joe was 19.

Joe joined the Marines at age 20 because he believed the structure of the military would be good for him and he wanted to be part of something meaningful. After completing boot camp, Joe was deployed to Afghanistan with his battalion. Although he had never smoked cigarettes before joining the military, Joe quickly adopted the habit after he became close with some fellow Marines who smoked. He would later say that some of the best moments of his deployment were spent getting to know his comrades while they smoked cigarettes during their down time.

Joe was frequently exposed to IED (improvised explosive device) explosions. During one blast he suffered a blow to the head, but he otherwise suffered no physical injuries during his time on active duty. One night Joe's battalion was ambushed when he was on patrol. During the course of the battle, Joe had to shoot multiple enemy soldiers, saw several friends injured or killed, and was certain he himself would die. To this day, Joe has few memories of the ambush, which is fine with him because he just wants to forget what happened.

Joe was deployed a total of three times over 3 years. He drank alcohol frequently and heavily on base between deployments, often to the point of "blacking out," and continued smoking cigarettes daily. When he finally returned to live with his family, his 4-year-old son did not remember him, and his wife had just given birth to their daughter.

Before Joe was deployed, he was an optimistic person who was usually in a good mood. After he returned from Afghanistan, however, Joe had a pessimistic outlook, both of himself and of the world. He believed that he was a bad person because of what he had done in battle, and he felt guilty that he had survived when others had not. He avoided watching the news because any discussion of the ongoing war brought back memories that made him angry. Joe recalled hearing that the local Veterans Administration Medical Center (VAMC) offered assistance to veterans who were having problems postdeployment. Although reluctant to go anywhere that reminded him of the military, Joe went to the VAMC emergency department, asking for help. He met with a psychiatrist and was diagnosed with an unspecified personality disorder and alcohol use disorder. Joe wanted help but felt anxious when he was asked questions about a prior trauma because this brought back distressing memories and uncomfortable feelings. He did not discuss his traumatic experiences and ended the interview abruptly.

Joe continued to be "moody" and was frequently irritated with his wife, their young son, and their new baby. He felt anxious and had trouble sleeping but discovered that the nights were more tolerable if he drank four to six beers before he went to bed. When he finally fell asleep, Joe had nightmares about the ambush and the friends he could not save. He soon discovered that a beer or two after waking up from a nightmare would allow him to go back to sleep for a few more restless hours.

Joe took the bus each day to and from his job at a local bank. The crowded space and loud traffic noises made him tense, and he constantly worried that something "bad" was about to happen. He spent the entire bus ride watching the doors and certain passengers who looked suspicious to him. After the evening bus trip home, he was even more anxious than when he left in the morning. Joe switched from drinking beer in the evenings to hard alcohol because beer no longer managed his anxiety as it did when he first started drinking. Every morning he would wake up well before his alarm went off with a racing heart, sweats, and a feeling of sheer panic. He drank coffee and smoked cigarettes throughout the work day to help manage anxiety, fatigue, and poor concentration. Sometimes he would get angry during a meeting and would walk out before it ended because he did not want to get into arguments with his co-workers.

At home, Joe often felt guilty because he was relatively healthy and still had his family while some of his friends, who also had families, had been killed. When he was not feeling guilty, he felt angry at the world because of what happened to him and others in Afghanistan. He had a hard time having fun with his family, and they did not enjoy spending time with him because they never knew what might make him angry.

Joe's friend introduced him to marijuana and he found he felt more relaxed after he smoked. He also began drinking larger amounts of hard alcohol because he discovered that the combination of marijuana and alcohol numbed his feelings of guilt, distanced him from his anger, and allowed him to fall asleep quickly. Over time, Joe began taking hits of marijuana during smoke breaks and drinking nip bottles of alcohol in the employee bathroom to help him manage fatigue as well as feelings of anger and anxiety at work.

When his wife started complaining about his use, Joe tried to stop smoking marijuana and cigarettes. Whenever he stopped smoking marijuana, however, he constantly thought about it and had a strong desire to use. Joe had a difficult time remaining abstinent for even a few hours at first. When he finally managed to stop smoking cannabis for a few days, he felt extremely agitated and could not fall asleep for several hours after he went to bed. He began drinking more and more hard alcohol to help him relax during the day and fall asleep at night.

Feeling unhappy and concerned that his marriage and job were in jeopardy, Joe presented to a VAMC emergency room again for help. He was sweaty and tremulous on presentation and his pulse was 113. He had an MCV of 102 and an AST/ALT ratio of 74/30. This time, he was admitted for detoxification from alcohol and subsequently diagnosed with PTSD. After starting naltrexone and engaging in an outpatient treatment program that addressed both PTSD and substance abuse, Joe was able to reduce his drinking and stop smoking marijuana, but he continued smoking cigarettes.

# Discussion

Joe experienced significant trauma during his deployment and subsequently developed PTSD. He reported *intrusion* symptoms (e.g., nightmares), *avoidance* of triggering stimuli (e.g., television reports that reminded him of combat, memories of the trauma), persistently *negative alterations in both cognitions and mood* (e.g., inability to remember parts of the traumatic event, persistent guilt), and *alterations in arousal and reactivity* (e.g., irritable behavior, sleep disturbances) (American Psychiatric Association 2013). He was formally diagnosed only after completing detoxification because PTSD assessments should not be conducted until patients are no longer in a state of intoxication or withdrawal (Ouimette and Brown 2003). The diagnosis of PTSD can be made with a clinical interview, but there are also several structured assessments, such as the Structured Clinical Interview for DSM Disorders (SCID) or the Clinician Administered PTSD Scale (CAPS), that can aid in making the diagnosis (Saladin et al. 2014). In reviewing Joe's history, it is clear that he had had several pretrauma risk factors for developing PTSD before he joined the Marines. These include lower socioeconomic status and history of early childhood trauma (American Psychiatric Association 2013). Additionally, Joe experienced what would be considered a severe trauma in the military because his life was threatened, his friends were injured or killed in front of him, and his defense of self and others resulted in the death of enemy fighters. All his combat experiences, coupled with his childhood experiences, increased his risk of developing PTSD (American Psychiatric Association 2013).

Given the high comorbidity between PTSD and SUDs (Table 5–3), when evaluating for one disorder, clinicians should always screen for the other. Furthermore, it has been suggested that PTSD is commonly underdiagnosed (Zimmerman and Mattia 1999). Conducting a sensitive interview with individuals who have experienced trauma is critical because discussing these events can be difficult and distressing for some individuals (MacKinnon et al. 2006). In Joe's case, he felt too uncomfortable when asked about trauma exposure when he first presented to the emergency room. His discomfort prevented him from answering these questions and the diagnosis of PTSD was missed.

For an accurate PTSD diagnosis in individuals who also abuse substances, it is important to consider the symptoms of substance intoxication and withdrawal that might overlap with PTSD symptoms (Table 5–2). Given that patients with PTSD are 80% more likely to have another psychiatric disorder compared with patients without PTSD, other psychiatric conditions should be also considered and either ruled out or treated accordingly (American Psychiatric Association 2013). Conditions in which symptoms must be distinguished from PTSD symptoms include anxiety, depressive, personality, dissociative, conversion, and psychotic disorders, as well as traumatic brain injury (TBI) (American Psychiatric Association 2013).

Joe's substance use, which started with social tobacco use when he was in the Marines, evolved into the use of several substances to help him manage PTSD symptoms. As Joe's PTSD symptoms worsened, he began using other substances and over time used them in larger amounts and with greater frequency. Indeed, drinking alcohol, smoking marijuana, and smoking cigarettes became Joe's self-prescribed "treatment" for PTSD. Joe soon found himself using these substances more than initially intended, needing more and more of these substances to manage his PTSD symptoms, and experiencing cravings just a few hours after his last use. Despite awareness of the problems his substance use was causing, Joe was unable to stop despite repeated attempts to quit. Ultimately, he needed to be admitted to the hospital because he could not decrease his alcohol use without experiencing withdrawal symptoms. By the time he entered treatment, Joe's signs and symptoms met criteria for alcohol, cannabis, and tobacco use disorders.

In the end, Joe was able to reduce his use of alcohol and stop smoking cannabis, but he continued to smoke cigarettes. This is not an unusual outcome, because individuals with PTSD who smoke cigarettes are more likely to be heavy smokers and are less likely to quit that those without PTSD (Fu et al. 2007). However, it has been suggested that patients with PTSD have quit rates comparable to those of smokers without a comorbid psychiatric diagnosis when engaged in smoking cessation treatment (Fu et al. 2007).

A medical evaluation of patients with PTSD and SUDs may be warranted, because having both disorders has been associated with more cardiovascular, neurological, and total chronic physical symptoms compared with individuals with SUDs alone (Ouimette et al. 2006). As with any patient where SUDs are part of the differential, individuals with PTSD and co-occurring SUDs should have basic laboratory tests (including complete blood count, general chemistries, and liver function tests) as well as urine toxicology screens. Veterans with comorbid PTSD and SUD have been shown to present with more symptoms of dependence, including a longer history of substance use, more social and legal problems, and more violent behaviors and suicide attempts (Young et al. 2005). Because of this, an assessment of the risk for suicide and violence is an important part of both the initial encounter and future clinical encounters. Furthermore, the presence of TBI complicates the treatment of PTSD and SUD, and in Joe's case, the blow to the head he suffered during his service requires assessment (Brady et al. 2009).

Over time, Joe's efforts to curb his PTSD symptoms by using different substances actually made some of his symptoms worse. It is important, therefore, to establish a timeline of PTSD symptom onset and to consider whether symptoms were improved or exacerbated by substance use. For example, Joe's sleeping problems, especially his nightmares, are clearly related to PTSD. Initial use of certain substances such as alcohol may allow patients with PTSD to fall asleep quickly, but more prolonged use can lead to more severe sleep problems, which, in turn, can lead to even more substance use (Vandrey et al. 2014). Joe's alcohol use allowed him to fall asleep quickly and to sleep through the night at first, but he eventually started to experience withdrawal symptoms early in the morning. He then began waking in the middle of the night and had to drink alcohol to manage withdrawal symptoms and go back to sleep. When he woke for the day, alcohol withdrawal symptoms such as palpitations, diaphoresis, and anxiety started even before he left his home for work. Similarly, marijuana use initially made him feel more relaxed, but soon he began feeling even more irritable on days when he did not smoke, a symptom of cannabis withdrawal (American Psychiatric Association 2013). Psychoeducation is important because patients may have limited insight into the connections among PTSD symptoms, substance use, and substance withdrawal.

There are different theories as to why PTSD and SUD commonly co-occur (Khantzian 1997; Saladin et al. 2014). According to the self-medication hypothesis, distressing symptoms of PTSD lead to substance use in an effort to minimize the untreated symptoms (Khantzian 1997). A second possibility is that people with SUDs are more likely to experience trauma because the lifestyle associated with using puts them in potentially dangerous situations, making traumatic experiences and the development of PTSD more likely (Saladin et al. 2014). A final theory is that the states of hyperarousal that are associated with intoxication or withdrawal states put people at physiological risk for developing PTSD upon exposure to traumatic events (Saladin et al. 2014). There is likely dysregulation of the hypothalamic-pituitary axis and noradrenergic systems that is common to both disorders (Jacobsen et al. 2001).

# Treatment

Individuals with PTSD and co-occurring SUDs are difficult to retain in treatment, have poor treatment outcomes, and have high relapse rates posttreatment (Weiss et al. 2004). Historically, the sequential treatment model was the mainstay of treatment. In this model, only the SUD would be treated at first and referral to PTSD treatment would occur after the individual successfully completed SUD treatment (Saladin et al. 2014). It was believed that achieving abstinence was the necessary first step before addressing PTSD, because the problems associated with active substance use prevented meaningful engagement in PTSD treatment. Additionally, there were concerns that the potential psychological distress that might arise when addressing trauma during PTSD treatment could put these dually diagnosed individuals at risk for relapse (Saladin et al. 2014). Others, however, have advocated for an integrated treatment model in which simultaneous treatment for both disorders is provided by the same treatment team in one treatment setting (Weiss et al. 2004).

To date, integrated treatment of PTSD and SUDs has been the primary focus in the research literature and has been shown to lead to improvements in both disorders (Saladin et al. 2014). Additionally, medications alone or in combination with psychotherapy show promise in the treatment of co-occurring PTSD and SUD. Below, we discuss specific psychosocial and psychopharmacological options for individuals with co-occurring PTSD and SUDs. See Table 5–4 for treatment tips.

## PSYCHOTHERAPEUTIC AND PSYCHOSOCIAL INTERVENTIONS

Psychotherapeutic and psychosocial interventions lie at the heart of the integrated treatment of co-occurring PTSD and SUDs. Several treatments have demonstrated particular effectiveness. *Seeking Safety* is the best-

**TABLE 5–4.  Treatment tips**

Individuals with posttraumatic stress disorder (PTSD) and substance use disorders (SUDs) can engage in integrated treatments, such as Seeking Safety and COPE, which address both disorders simultaneously without experiencing worsening of either disorder.

12-step program involvement may be most appropriate for those who identify with the 12-step philosophy.

Sertraline may be an appropriate medication for individuals whose PTSD develops before alcohol use disorder.

Naltrexone and disulfiram are appropriate medications for treating alcohol use disorder when it co-occurs with PTSD. Disulfiram may also help reduce symptoms of PTSD.

Treating opioid dependence with methadone or buprenorphine in individuals with PTSD can reduce substance use and help break the cycle of addiction.

known integrated cognitive-behavioral therapy (CBT) for co-occurring PTSD and SUDs (Najavitis 2002), and it would be an appropriate treatment for Joe. The goal of this structured, manualized therapy is to reduce symptoms of co-occurring PTSD and SUDs by helping patients understand and explore the relationship between the disorders and teaching healthy coping skills for both. The treatment is divided into 25 sessions that address interpersonal, behavioral, cognitive, and case management topics and can be delivered by clinicians of various mental health degrees and clinical backgrounds. Topics in the manual include "PTSD: Taking Your Power Back," "When Substances Control You," "Coping with Triggers," "Healthy Relationships," and "Self-Nurturing." Although originally developed as a group treatment for women, Seeking Safety has been adapted to treat men and adolescents in group settings, as well as individual patients. Studies of Seeking Safety have shown that it is effective in reducing substance use and improving PTSD symptoms (Najavitis 2002).

Treatment that integrates prolonged exposure therapy, a recommended treatment for PTSD, with CBT has also been described for individuals with co-occurring PTSD and SUDs (Brady et al. 2001; Mills et al. 2012). Prolonged exposure therapy for PTSD involves psychoeducation about common reactions to traumatic events, relaxation exercises, prolonged imaginal exposure to the trauma by a therapist-guided retelling of the trauma, and in vivo exposure to trauma-related situations that the individual avoids because of fear (Saladin et al. 2014). Initially developed as a concurrent treatment for PTSD and cocaine dependence (Back et al.

2001), the integrated prolonged exposure therapy and CBT model was later modified to include other SUDs (Mills et al. 2012), and this would also be a treatment option for Joe. *Concurrent Treatment of PTSD and Substance Use Disorders using Prolonged Exposure*, more commonly known as COPE, is delivered individually over 13 sessions and includes motivational enhancement and CBT for substance use, psychoeducation about both disorders and their interaction, in vivo exposure, imaginal exposure, and CBT for PTSD (Mills et al. 2012). When combined with usual substance abuse treatment found in the community (i.e., outpatient counseling, detoxification, residential programs, and medications for SUDs), COPE was associated with improvements in PTSD symptoms. Although substance use did not improve among subjects, substance use also did not increase, which is a common concern when individuals with SUDs enter prolonged exposure treatment (Mills et al. 2012).

The appropriateness of 12-step programs such as Alcoholics Anonymous for individuals with PTSD and comorbid PTSD has been a subject of debate. It has been suggested that these dually diagnosed individuals may have a hard time affiliating with 12-step programs because they may view their PTSD as the primary problem while the other 12-step group members may encourage them to view their SUD as primary (Satel et al. 1993). Additionally, it is thought that they may have difficulty connecting with other group members because of a desire to avoid close relationships with other people. One study, however, showed that greater participation in 12-step activities was associated with decreased psychological distress among individuals with co-occurring PTSD and SUD who identified with the 12-step philosophy, while the opposite was true for those who did not identify with the 12-step philosophy (Ouimette et al. 2001). Twelve-step groups can be an important component of treatment for PTSD and SUDs, but it is important for the clinician to evaluate a patient's conceptualization of their PTSD and SUD before encouraging 12-step involvement.

At present, other treatments for PTSD, such as eye movement desensitization and reprocessing (EMDR), biofeedback, and stress inoculation training, have not been studied for those with co-occurring PTSD and SUDs.

## PHARMACOLOGICAL INTERVENTIONS

Studies have shown that several medications may be helpful for people with co-occurring PTSD and SUDs. Two separate studies have examined sertraline, a U.S. Food and Drug Administration (FDA)–approved medication for PTSD, for the treatment of co-occurring PTSD and alcohol dependence (Brady et al. 1995, 2005). These studies found that the medication reduced alcohol use and symptoms of PTSD during 12 weeks of treatment. Interestingly, sertraline was associated with a greater reduction in the number of drinks consumed per drinking day for those individuals with less severe alcohol dependence who developed PTSD prior to development of their alcohol dependence (i.e., primary PTSD) (Brady et al. 2005). These studies imply that patients with primary PTSD and secondary alcohol dependence might respond preferentially to antidepressant medication compared with those whose alcohol dependence predated the onset of PTSD (Brady et al. 2005). Since Joe experienced trauma and developed PTSD symptoms prior to heavy drinking, sertraline could be an appropriate medication to treat both disorders.

Naltrexone and disulfiram, two FDA-approved medications for alcohol use disorder, may also be effective treatments for co-occurring PTSD and alcohol dependence. In one study, the effects of placebo, naltrexone only, disulfiram only, and naltrexone and disulfiram combined were examined in a group of veterans with alcohol dependence (Petrakis et al. 2006). In a subgroup of veterans with comorbid PTSD, all three medication conditions were associated with greater number of days abstinent and greater reductions in the number of heavy drinking days compared with placebo. Additionally, disulfiram was associated with greater reductions in total scores on the Clinician-Administered PTSD Scale (CAPS) when compared with naltrexone and placebo. In addition to its typical impact on alcohol use, which may improve PTSD symptoms, reduction of adrenergic activity secondary to disulfiram's inhibition of the enzyme dopamine beta-hydroxylase, which leads to an increase in central nervous system dopamine and a reduction in norepinephrine synthesis, was hypothesized as a reason for PTSD symptom reduction (Petrakis et al. 2006).

It has been suggested that there are two discrete groups of individuals with PTSD and opioid use disorder (Shorter et al. 2015). The first comprises those who are dependent on opioids, experience a trauma, and then develop PTSD. The second are those who experience a trauma and, after being treated with opioids, develop an opioid use disorder. In either scenario, it appears that treatment with opioid replacement therapies such as methadone and buprenorphine can help stop the cycle of addiction and improve overall quality of life. Although no studies have examined the effectiveness of opioid replacement therapies for individuals with PTSD and comorbid opioid use disorder, one study showed that opioid antagonists reduced substance use equally in those with PTSD and those without a co-occurring psychiatric diagnosis (Trafton et al. 2006).

One study did examine the combination of naltrexone and psychotherapy for individuals with both PTSD and alcohol dependence (Foa et al. 2013). Naltrexone appeared to reduce the total number of drinking days in patients who received either of the active therapies (prolonged exposure, which is the standard PTSD treatment, and supportive psychotherapy, which is viewed as suboptimal in this population) when compared with placebo. PTSD symptoms were similarly reduced among all active treatment conditions. By 6-month follow-up, those in the combined naltrexone–prolonged exposure group had relapsed to alcohol use at a lower rate than the other study groups.

At present, there are no pharmacological studies of the treatment of PTSD and co-occurring cocaine, cannabis, tobacco, or sedative-hypnotic dependence.

# Conclusion

PTSD and SUDs commonly occur and are often underdiagnosed and undertreated. As was seen in the case of Joe, many patients with co-occurring disorders develop SUDs after developing PTSD. In other situations, persons with SUDs who experience trauma have an elevated risk of developing PTSD. Regardless of the order in which an individual develops these disorders, it is critical that both disorders be addressed simultaneously with psychosocial interventions and psychotropic medications to obtain the best treatment outcomes.

## KEY POINTS

- Individuals with posttraumatic stress disorder (PTSD) are at greater risk of developing substance use disorders (SUDs), and individuals with SUDs are at an increased risk of experiencing trauma and developing PTSD.

- Integrated treatments for PTSD and SUDs, such as Seeking Safety and COPE, as well as pharmacological interventions, have been shown to be effective for treating these disorders when they co-occur.

- Involvement in 12-step programs may decrease distress in individuals with co-occurring PTSD and SUDs who identify with the 12-step philosophy.

# Questions

1.  Which of the following psychosocial approaches treats posttrau-
    matic stress disorder (PTSD) and substance use disorders (SUDs)
    by addressing such topics as "Coping with Triggers" and "Self-
    Nurturing"?

    A. Alcoholics Anonymous.
    B. Biofeedback.
    C. Seeking Safety.
    D. Eye movement desensitization and reprocessing (EMDR).

2.  Which of the following medications may be most effective for those
    individuals who develop PTSD prior to alcohol dependence?

    A. Sertraline.
    B. Naltrexone.
    C. Buprenorphine.
    D. Paroxetine.

3.  Which of the following is *true* about the evaluation of an individual
    with PTSD and a SUD?

    A. A clinician can avoid questions about legal problems, because
       they are uncommon in individuals with PTSD and SUDs.
    B. When an individual presents with symptoms of intoxication
       or withdrawal from a substance, he or she should not be im-
       mediately evaluated for PTSD.
    C. Rarely are issues with smoking and smoking cessation encoun-
       tered in individuals with PTSD and SUDs.
    D. A clinician should focus, in the evaluation, on trauma that has
       occurred when individuals were not using substances.

# References

American Psychiatric Association: Diagnostic and Statistical Manual of Mental
    Disorders, 5th Edition. Arlington, VA, American Psychiatric Association,
    2013
Back SE, Dansky BS, Carroll KM, et al: Exposure therapy in the treatment of
    PTSD among cocaine-dependent individuals: description of procedures.
    J Subst Abuse Treat 21(1):35–45, 2001 11516925

Brady KT, Sonne SC, Roberts JM: Sertraline treatment of comorbid posttraumatic stress disorder and alcohol dependence. J Clin Psychiatry 56(11):502–505, 1995 7592501

Brady KT, Dansky BS, Back SE, et al: Exposure therapy in the treatment of PTSD among cocaine-dependent individuals: preliminary findings. J Subst Abuse Treat 21(1):47–54, 2001 11516926

Brady KT, Sonne S, Anton RF, et al: Sertraline in the treatment of co-occurring alcohol dependence and posttraumatic stress disorder. Alcohol Clin Exp Res 29:395–401, 2005 15770115

Brady KT, Tuerk P, Back SE, et al: Combat posttraumatic stress disorder, substance use disorders, and traumatic brain injury. J Addict Med 3(4):179–188, 2009 21769015

Foa EB, Yusko DA, McLean CP, et al: Concurrent naltrexone and prolonged exposure therapy for patients with comorbid alcohol dependence and PTSD: a randomized clinical trial. JAMA 310(5):488–495, 2013 23925619

Fu SS, McFall M, Saxon AJ, et al: Post-traumatic stress disorder and smoking: a systematic review. Nicotine Tob Res 9(11):1071–1084, 2007 17978982

Jacobsen LK, Southwick SM, Kosten TR: Substance use disorders in patients with posttraumatic stress disorder: a review of the literature. Am J Psychiatry 158(8):1184–1190, 2001 11481147

Kessler RC, Sonnega A, Bromet E, et al: Posttraumatic stress disorder in the National Comorbidity Survey. Arch Gen Psychiatry 52(12):1048–1060, 1995 7492257

Khantzian EJ: The self-medication hypothesis of substance use disorders: a reconsideration and recent applications. Harv Rev Psychiatry 4(5):231–244, 1997 9385000

MacKinnon RA, Michels R, Buckley PJ: The Psychiatric Interview in Clinical Practice, 2nd Edition. Washington, DC, American Psychiatric Publishing, 2006

Mills KL, Teesson M, Back SE, et al: Integrated exposure-based therapy for co-occurring posttraumatic stress disorder and substance dependence: a randomized controlled trial. JAMA 308(7):690–699, 2012 22893166

Najavitis L: Seeking Safety: A Treatment Manual for PTSD and Substance Abuse. New York, Guilford, 2002

Ouimette P, Brown PJ: Trauma and Substance Abuse: Causes, Consequences, and Treatment of Comorbid Disorders. Washington, DC, American Psychological Association, 2003

Ouimette P, Humphreys K, Moos RH, et al: Self-help group participation among substance use disorder patients with posttraumatic stress disorder. J Subst Abuse Treat 20(1):25–32, 2001 11239725

Ouimette P, Goodwin E, Brown PJ: Health and well being of substance use disorder patients with and without posttraumatic stress disorder. Addict Behav 31(8):1415–1423, 2006 16380217

Petrakis IL, Poling J, Levinson C, et al: Naltrexone and disulfiram in patients with alcohol dependence and comorbid post-traumatic stress disorder. Biol Psychiatry 60(7):777–783, 2006 17008146

Reynolds M, Mezey G, Chapman M, et al: Co-morbid post-traumatic stress disorder in a substance misusing population. Drug Alcohol Depend 77:251–258, 2005 15734225

Saladin ME, Back SE, Payne RA, et al: Posttraumatic stress disorder and substance use disorder comorbidity, in The ASAM Principles of Addiction Medicine. Edited by Ries RK, Fiellin DA, Miller SC, et al. Philadelphia, PA, Lippincott Williams & Wilkins, 2014, pp 1403–1417

Satel SL, Becker BR, Dan E: Reducing obstacles to affiliation with alcoholics anonymous among veterans with PTSD and alcoholism. Hosp Community Psychiatry 44(11):1061–1065, 1993 8288174

Schäfer I, Najavits LM: Clinical challenges in the treatment of patients with posttraumatic stress disorder and substance abuse. Curr Opin Psychiatry 20(6):614–618, 2007 17921765

Shorter D, Hsieh J, Kosten TR: Pharmacologic management of comorbid posttraumatic stress disorder and addictions. Am J Addict 24(8):705–712, 2015 26587796

Trafton JA, Minkel J, Humphreys K: Opioid substitution treatment reduces substance use equivalently in patients with and without posttraumatic stress disorder. J Stud Alcohol 67(2):228–235, 2006 16562404

Vandrey R, Babson KA, Herrmann ES, Bonn-Miller MO: Interactions between disordered sleep, post-traumatic stress disorder, and substance use disorders. Int Rev Psychiatry 26(2):237–247, 2014 24892898

Weiss RD, Najavitis LM, Hennessy G: Overview of treatment modalities for dual-diagnosis patients: pharmacotherapy, psychotherapy, and 12-step programs, in Dual Diagnosis and Psychiatric Treatment: Substance Abuse and Psychiatric Disorders, 2nd Edition. Edited by Kranzler HR, Tinsley J. New York, Marcel Dekker, 2004, pp 103–128

Young HE, Rosen CS, Finney JW: A survey of PTSD screening and referral practices in VA addiction treatment programs. J Subst Abuse Treat 28(4):313–319, 2005 15925265

Zimmerman M, Mattia JI: Is posttraumatic stress disorder underdiagnosed in routine clinical settings? J Nerv Ment Dis 187(7):420–428, 1999 10426462

# 6

# PSYCHOTIC DISORDERS

*Bernadine H. Han, M.D., M.S.*
*Jonathan D. Avery, M.D.*

Patients often present with psychosis and evidence of substance use disorders (SUDs), and treating these individuals is often challenging. Ideal treatment addresses both conditions simultaneously with psychosocial and pharmacological interventions.

Many of these patients develop psychoses after using psychoactive substances such as phencyclidine (PCP), cannabis, or stimulants. Other patients may develop psychotic symptoms as part of a delirium in the context of an acute withdrawal from alcohol or benzodiazepines (Table 6–1). Still others might present with acute psychotic symptoms that stem from both a primary psychotic disorder and the effect of a psychoactive substance (Table 6–2).

Actively addressing all relevant diagnoses is central to the effective treatment of patients with co-occurring psychosis and SUDs. SUDs are common among people with schizophrenia, for example, but treatments usually focus only on the schizophrenia. This may reflect greater concern about the symptoms and debilitation caused by schizophrenia, or the perception that treating SUDs in chronically psychotic patients is too

**TABLE 6–1.** Overview of substance-induced psychotic symptoms

| Substance | Intoxication/ withdrawal | Effect | Treatment |
|---|---|---|---|
| Alcohol/ benzodiazepine | Withdrawal | Auditory and visual hallucinations, initially with otherwise clear mental status. Increasing agitation | Benzodiazepines, per withdrawal guidelines<br>Antipsychotics for agitation |
| Cannabis | Intoxication | Paranoid delusions, and auditory/ visual hallucinations, may be affectively tinged. Chronic use associated with primary psychotic disorder | Symptomatic with antipsychotics and/or benzodiazepines |
| Cocaine | Intoxication | Paranoia, auditory/visual/tactile hallucinations. Greater risk with heavy regular use, younger patients | Symptomatic with antipsychotics and/or benzodiazepines |
| Amphetamines | Intoxication | Paranoia, ideas of reference, persecutory delusions, auditory/ visual hallucinations, agitation | Benzodiazepines to sedate<br>Avoid chlorpromazine for compounded risk of lowered seizure threshold |
| Hallucinogens | Intoxication | Paranoia, aggression | Benzodiazepines<br>Antipsychotics prn |
| PCP, ketamine, dextromethorphan | Intoxication | Dissociation, anesthesia; severe aggression, violence, and paranoia with PCP | Benzodiazepines to sedate<br>High-potency, low-anticholinergic antipsychotics like haloperidol prn |
| MDMA (ecstasy) | Intoxication | Mixed mood/anxiety/psychotic symptoms | Benzodiazepines |

*Note.*   MDMA=3,4-methylenedioxy-methamphetamine; PCP=phencyclidine.

**TABLE 6–2.** Common co-occurring substance use disorders (SUDs) with schizophrenia

| SUD | Percentage of schizophrenia patients with this SUD |
|---|---|
| Nicotine | 70%–90% |
| Alcohol | 34% |
| Drug use disorder | 28% |
| Cocaine | 16% |
| Cannabis | 6% |

*Source.* Ziedonis et al. 2014.

difficult. From our perspective, however, it is important to identify and treat SUDs in this vulnerable population while treating the schizophrenia. Ideally, an integrated treatment would involve antipsychotic medications, psychosocial intervention, targeted psychotherapy, and SUD treatments that accommodate the functional and cognitive limitations often found in people with schizophrenia.

In the following case, we describe a young woman who presents with psychotic symptoms in the setting of heavy marijuana use. We then discuss her evaluation and treatment, as well as more general treatment options for individuals with co-occurring psychosis and substance use disorders.

## Clinical Case

Jessi is a 23-year-old woman who was brought to the outpatient psychiatric clinic by her mother after she had experienced at least several months of psychotic symptoms, 2 years of declining social and academic functioning, and at least 3 years of daily marijuana use. Jessi had never previously seen a mental health professional and had never received a formal medical or psychiatric diagnosis. Family history was pertinent for schizophrenia in the maternal grandfather.

Jessi and her mother report she began to use marijuana daily when she started college to "fit in" and to "self-medicate" her anxiety. In high school, she did well academically in the classes that she liked, barely passed a few of her classes, and had few friends. She found that marijuana helped her find a group of peers and "relax" in the new environment. After receiving A's and B's in her first two years of college, her grades steadily declined, and she was barely able to graduate. Instead of studying or attending class, which she felt to be irrelevant, she spent her time on a series of online startup businesses. She reports that each of her business ideas failed because someone had figured out her idea and "beaten her to the punch."

She has lived with her mother since graduation. She spends her days online or playing video games. While she would smoke marijuana with her roommates in college, she now uses alone, from the time she wakes up until she goes to bed.

In recent months, she has spent all of her time on her latest start-up project, which she describes as "top-secret." Unlike her previous efforts, she does not want to let anyone know about her ideas, because "many people would like to steal them." She has had her mother taste her food just in case anyone "tries to do her in secretly." Her mother has heard her from her room talking to herself about "unlocking the key to capitalism."

Jessi does not feel like she needs any help and has no desire to cut down on her marijuana use or to engage in mental health treatment. She denies all current mood and anxiety symptoms and any thoughts to harm herself or others. Her mother is hopeful that she will cut down on her marijuana use and try medications that will help to bring her "old daughter" back.

Jessi also smokes 1 pack per day of tobacco. She denies alcohol use and other illicit substances. A toxicology screen was positive only for cannabis. Routine labs revealed a normal MCV and AST/ALT. Head imaging was normal. HIV test was negative.

# Discussion

Upon her initial presentation, Jessi has a clear marijuana use disorder, in which her marijuana use is implicated in her poor functioning. Her psychotic symptoms appear to have developed in the context of the heavy marijuana use, and marijuana is known to induce psychosis. Her initial diagnosis would, therefore, include both the marijuana use disorder and a marijuana-induced psychotic disorder.

The underlying etiology of the psychosis is, however, uncertain, and the differential diagnosis would also include a primary psychotic disorder such as schizophrenia; bipolar disorder with psychotic features (the grandiosity would suggest possible mania); and a psychosis secondary to a medical condition. For the primary psychotic disorder to be diagnosed, the patient would have to remain psychotic after at least a month's abstinence from the marijuana. DSM-5 asks the clinician to use judgment in regard to the necessary duration of abstinence, and the duration varies between people and between substances. For example, people tend to clear from the depression of cocaine withdrawal within a few days, whereas the psychotic reaction to synthetic cannabinoids and methamphetamine can last for months after their discontinuation (Ziedonis et al. 2014).

As is often the case in real-world situations, however, the clinician is meeting with a patient who has not had a recent episode of abstinence and is demonstrating minimal motivation to discontinue her substance of abuse. Although DSM-5 would suggest we defer making a primary psychiatric diagnosis until this patient has been abstinent for about a month, we can still consider possibilities. For example, schizophrenia would be a serious possibility, and we know that cannabis has a strong relationship to schizophrenia. For example, cannabis use correlates with earlier onset of schizophrenia, increased lifetime risk of psychosis, and increased risk of psychotic episodes after initial treatment and remission of symptoms (Ziedonis et al. 2014). At the same time, studies show that in cases of substance-induced psychosis, only 1%–15% of patients still have symptoms after one month of abstinence (Ziedonis et al. 2014), so Jessi might improve significantly if her SUD is effectively treated.

The workup for someone with co-occurring psychosis and substance use would be similar to the workup of anyone with either of these diagnoses.

Thyroid or cortisol-related conditions (including steroid treatment), deliriogenic metabolic conditions (including hypoxia, hypercarbia, hypoglycemia, and water and salt imbalance), end-stage organ disease of the liver or kidneys, and autoimmune or metastatic processes affecting the brain are among the many medical conditions to consider in a suspected organic cause of acute psychotic symptoms (Ziedonis et al. 2014).

In other words, patients presenting with psychosis and a SUD would typically get routine bloodwork (metabolic panel, complete blood count, thyroid function tests) as well as screens for alcohol and illicit substances. A general physical and neurological exam should be done; head scans are generally negative unless an abnormality is detected on the physical or neurological exams, but most protocols would still include a head scan for a new-onset psychosis.

Collateral information can be as important to an accurate diagnosis as the mental status exam and overall clinical presentation. While talking to friends and family or while reviewing available records, the clinician will try to clarify the patient's history of substance use, previous psychiatric history, response to treatment efforts, and outside support systems. Initial history elicited from a close contact may also contribute to the treatment phase. In Jessi's case, for example, it will be useful to engage the mother in the efforts to assess continued use during a diagnostic period. Such efforts from collateral sources are important, since both psychosis and substance use may diminish a patient's ability or willingness to accurately report substance use.

Even when the diagnosis is uncertain, a prolonged diagnostic period must not preclude or delay adequate treatment for both suspected conditions. This need for treatment during this period is supported by studies showing that about 25% of patients initially diagnosed with psychosis secondary to substance use will later receive a diagnosis of a primary psychotic disorder (Ziedonis et al. 2014).

A number of theories exist as to why substance use disorders and psychotic disorders have a high rate of concurrence. These theories tend to make intuitive sense (i.e., they tend to have "face validity"), but evidence is limited (Green et al. 2007). The stress-diathesis model suggests that substances may provide the adequate (and unfortunate) stress to trigger a genetic vulnerability toward psychosis. The presence of schizophrenia in Jessi's grandfather, for example, suggests she may have some genetic tendency toward schizophrenia but that the marijuana may have been involved in some way with the timing or severity of the psychotic symptoms (Green et al. 2007). The reverse possibility—that patients with psychotic disorder have a greater biological sensitivity to substance effects and greater potential for substance abuse—has also been suggested (Green et al. 2007). It is also possible that Jessi's grandfather's "schizophrenia" was actually undiagnosed bipolar disorder or substance use disorder rather than schizophrenia and that Jessi inherited a genetic tendency toward one of those disorders.

Another consideration is that a psychotic illness can contribute to the accumulation of risk factors for substance use, such as impaired cognition, less education, unemployment, and decreased social function, and residence in challenging social environments (Green et al. 2007). The typical age at onset of schizophrenia and bipolar disorder—late adolescence or young adulthood—corresponds with the typical initial age at onset of drug experimentation; substance use during early psychosis can lead to a comforting sense that the patient is in control of his of her disturbing symptoms. Becoming part of a substance-using social group can also contribute to the patient's sense of normalcy when, otherwise, his or her increasing impairment and oddity might be more obvious and upsetting.

Patients, themselves, often indicate that they use substances to self-medicate—to calm themselves, decrease anxiety, or escape their symptoms (Khantzian 1997). Jessi indicates that she used marijuana initially for "anxiety," but we do not know if she means an uneasy sense that she is becoming psychotic (which might point toward schizophrenia) or the desperate insomnia that can be part of bipolar disorder. Jessi may also have been trying to extend the effects of bipolar mania, since the intense, grandiose sense of apparent achievement may be more acceptable to her than the sluggishness of depression and the reality of mental illness. While it is tempting to consider possibilities, a better understanding of Jessi awaits her abstinence.

There are multiple biological theories that try to explain self-medication using the known effects of different substances on reward and anxiety pathways (Green et al. 2007; Khantzian 1997). In our case, Jessi described first using marijuana to help with anxiety. Substance use tends to change reward circuitry in everyone, but this may be especially pertinent in patients with co-occurring schizophrenia, in which there tends to be dysfunctional transmission along the dopamine reward pathway (Green et al. 2007; Ziedonis et al. 2014). In patients with schizophrenia, therefore, substance use may amplify the reward signals that may be impaired by the primary psychotic illness (Green et al. 2007; Ziedonis et al. 2014).

There are many real-life barriers to developing an effective diagnosis and appropriate treatment for patients with co-occurring substance use and psychotic disorders. Individuals with these disorders often have little insight into their condition, offer an incomplete history, deny the need for treatment, and do things that frustrate the best of psychiatric interventions (Avery and Zerbo 2015; Avery et al. 2016). Limited resources within a community and suboptimal insurance coverage may conspire to make thoughtful, integrated treatment challenging as well. At the same time, however, there have been many advances in our understanding on how to best treat these individuals.

# Treatment

Integrated treatment is important for patients with co-occurring psychotic disorders and SUDs. This perspective has been the standard since 2002, when a major governmental report concluded that integrated treatment leads to decreased substance use, reduced addiction severity, and fewer positive symptoms of psychosis compared with nonintegrated treatments (Green et al. 2007; Ziedonis et al. 2014). This report also

---

**TABLE 6–3. Treatment tips**

Individuals with psychosis can still benefit from psychosocial interventions for substance use disorders, including 12-step groups.

Second-generation antipsychotics may be more effective than first-generation antipsychotics for psychotic symptoms and substance use outcomes.

Cigarettes and caffeine use patterns will impact medication level.

The risk of worsening psychosis with disulfiram, varenicline, and other medications that target substance use is small.

---

directly led to enhanced Congressional funding of integrated treatment programs (Ziedonis et al. 2014). Nevertheless, clinicians continue to experience a lack of readily available treatment options for a population of patients that tends to dismiss the treatment that is offered (Avery and Zerbo 2015; Avery et al. 2016). While these realities can lead to a therapeutic nihilism, studies show that remission from substances like marijuana after a first-break psychosis is associated with better functional and social outcomes in long-term follow-up, even with the chronicity and recurrence of psychosis (Ziedonis et al. 2014).

Below we discuss specific psychosocial and psychopharmacological options for individuals with co-occurring psychotic disorders and SUDs. See Table 6–3 for treatment tips.

## PSYCHOTHERAPEUTIC AND PSYCHOSOCIAL INTERVENTIONS

As with Jessi and all patients who use substances, engagement in treatment is the first and arguably most challenging hurdle in receiving care (Avery and Zerbo 2015; Avery et al. 2016). Essential to engagement is the development of a nurturing and nonjudgmental therapeutic alliance in which the treater conveys hope for the future and confronts the reality of continued use (Ziedonis et al. 2014). From there, buy-in and commitment can be developed with therapies such as motivational enhancement therapy (MET) and motivational interviewing (see Chapter 12, "Motivational Interviewing").

Group therapy utilizing cognitive-behavioral therapy (CBT) and MET has been shown to be an effective psychotherapeutic approach in the treatment of SUDs with comorbid schizophrenia (Green et al. 2007; Ziedonis et al. 2014). CBT approaches often require modifications for the cognitive deficits, poor interpersonal skills, and low motivation associated with schizophrenia (Ziedonis et al. 2014). Likewise, motivation-based dual diagnosis treatment modifies the traditional motivational interviewing approach for patients with concurrent psychotic illness, creating a more active and ongoing role for the clinician (Ziedonis et al. 2014).

Alcoholics Anonymous and other 12-step groups may not be ideal for acutely psychotic patients. Dual Recovery Anonymous, however, often referred to as "Double Trouble," is a 12-step program that caters toward individuals with co-occurring mental illness and SUDs. It may appeal to patients who are willing to work within the 12-step model (Ziedonis et al. 2014).

It is useful to recognize that chronic psychotic illness is often accompanied by cognitive deficits. In patients who tend to be concrete or to have limited cognitive capacities and/or diminished executive functioning, it may be useful to emphasize therapeutic approaches that feature practical motivators such as external rewards and consequences. For example, contingency management involves giving patients tangible rewards to reinforce positive behaviors and appears to be useful in this patient population (Ziedonis et al. 2014). Relapse prevention and other approaches that incorporate behavioral rehearsal and role-playing, case management, and patient education all show improved outcomes versus treatment without these supports (Ziedonis et al. 2014).

Assertive case treatment, or ACT, is one example of an intensive outpatient service that can provide additional housing and advocacy services. These psychosocial and practical interventions have also been associated with greater abstinence (Ziedonis et al. 2014).

## PHARMACOLOGICAL INTERVENTIONS

When acute withdrawal/intoxication is controlled (see Table 6–1), and it is determined that an individual has both a psychotic disorder and a co-occurring SUD, the first goal of pharmacological treatment is to target psychotic symptoms. Adherence is often poor among patients with both substance and psychotic disorders but can improve with better psychotic symptom management, psychoeducation, MET, and skills training around medication management, as discussed earlier. Long-acting intramuscular injections of antipsychotic medication may be particularly useful in improving adherence for some patients.

There is fair evidence that second-generation antipsychotics (SGAs) for patients with co-occurring psychotic disorder and SUD, in addition to treating psychotic symptoms, increase abstinence and decrease craving in nicotine, alcohol, cannabis, and cocaine use disorders (Green et al. 2007; Murthy and Chand 2012; Ziedonis et al. 2014). Clozapine is especially effective at decreasing use of substances by up to 70%–80%, and these effects appear to be sustained long-term (Green et al. 2007; Mesholam-Gately et al. 2014; Murthy and Chand 2012; Ziedonis et al. 2014). First-generation antipsychotics (FGAs) do not have the same effect on substance use, and they may even worsen substance use (Green et al. 2007; Murthy and Chand 2012; Ziedonis et al. 2014). It should be noted that patients with SUDs without concurrent psychotic illness seem to have higher rates of akathisia and extrapyramidal symptoms than patients with schizophrenia alone, suggesting that patients with SUDs are at risk of worsened movement disorders with antipsychotic treatment (Green et al. 2007; Murthy and Chand 2012).

Most substances of abuse (as well as natural rewards, like food or sex) affect the mesolimbic circuit by ultimately increasing the amount of dopamine and the duration of its presence at the postsynaptic dopamine receptors in this pathway (Adinoff 2004). Antipsychotic medications antagonize this postsynaptic receptor, which may attenuate the reward sensation previously associated with use and perhaps, thereby reducing cravings (Adinoff 2004; Ziedonis et al. 2014). SGAs also have effects on serotonin, which may play a role in craving, and this may explain their superiority over FGAs (Green et al. 2007; Murthy and Chand 2012; Ziedonis et al. 2014). It is thought that clozapine's particular effects on serotonin receptors, in addition to norepinephrine and dopamine ($D_2$) receptors, account for its effectiveness in modulating the reward deficiency (Green et al. 2007; Murthy and Chand 2012).

Bupropion, varenicline, and nicotine replacement treatments may help with the tobacco use disorders that commonly co-occur in this population. As a dopamine agonist, bupropion may theoretically increase the risk of psychosis, but a recent systematic review showed minimal risk when weighed against the number of patients who benefited from it (Englisch et al. 2013). It is important to keep in mind that byproducts of tobacco smoking induce cytochrome P450 1A2 and thus may decrease levels of antipsychotics such as clozapine, olanzapine, and haloperidol (Ziedonis et al. 2014). Smokers tend to be on increased doses of antipsychotic medications compared with nonsmokers, and this can be clinically important with patients who are trying to quit or even those who are transitioning back to the community (and their cigarettes) after an extended inpatient admission.

Disulfiram, acamprosate, topiramate, and naltrexone are effective medications in alcohol use disorders. Although not much data exist for use of these agents in individuals with psychotic disorders, they are commonly and effectively prescribed. Possibly because of its inhibition of dopamine-β-hydroxylase, disulfiram seems to slightly increase the risk of dose-dependent psychosis, especially among patients with a personal or family history of psychotic symptoms (de Melo et al. 2014). The increased risk among patients with comorbid psychotic disorders warrants increased observation when these agents are being initiated and the dosage is being increased (de Melo et al. 2014).

Research on effective psychopharmacological treatments for cocaine, cannabis, and other drug use disorders comorbid with psychotic disorders is lacking. Despite that, just as with tobacco and alcohol use disorders, simultaneous treatment for both psychosis and substance use is recommended.

# Conclusion

Substance use disorders are common among individuals with psychotic spectrum disorders that include schizophrenia as well as the substance-induced psychosis. The case of Jessi illustrated a common presentation of such an individual. The treatment of these individuals is often challenging. Ideal treatment addresses both conditions simultaneously with psychosocial and psychopharmacological interventions.

## KEY POINTS

- About half of all patients with a primary psychotic disorder have a concurrent substance use disorder (SUD).

- In the majority of patients with co-occurring psychotic disorder and SUD(s), the substance use is undertreated, leading to worse outcomes and poorer control of psychotic symptoms.

- In patients with co-occurring psychotic disorder and SUD(s), treatments that integrate the management of both disorders (with pharmacological, psychotherapeutic, and psychosocial approaches) have been shown to be most effective at improving outcomes.

# Questions

1. Which of the following psychosocial approaches has not had consistently strong evidence in decreasing substance use among patients with schizophrenia and substance use disorders?

    A. Cognitive-behavioral therapy (CBT).

    B. Dual Recovery Anonymous (aka "Double Trouble").

    C. Motivational enhancement therapy (MET).

    D. Contingency management.

2. Which medication used in patients with concurrent chronic psychotic illness and substance use disorder has been shown to be most effective in reducing substance use and increasing abstinence?

    A. Haloperidol.

    B. Olanzapine.

    C. Clozapine.

    D. Bupropion.

3. Which are the three most commonly used substances among patients with concurrent psychotic and substance use disorders?

    A. Alcohol, cocaine, marijuana.

    B. Alcohol, cocaine, nicotine.

    C. Cocaine, marijuana, nicotine.

    D. Alcohol, marijuana, nicotine.

# References

Adinoff B: Neurobiologic processes in drug reward and addiction. Harv Rev Psychiatry 12(6):305–320, 2004 15764467

Avery J, Zerbo E: Improving psychiatry residents' attitudes toward individuals diagnosed with substance use disorders. Harv Rev Psychiatry 23(4):296–300, 2015 26146757

Avery J, Zerbo E, Ross S: Improving psychiatrists' attitudes towards individuals with psychotic disorders and co-occurring substance use disorders. Acad Psychiatry 40(3):520–522, 2016 25977100

de Melo RC, Lopes R, Alves JC: A case of psychosis in disulfiram treatment for alcoholism. Case Report Psychiatry 2014:561092, 2014 24818034

Englisch S, Morgen K, Meyer-Lindenberg A, Zink M: Risks and benefits of bupropion treatment in schizophrenia: a systematic review of the current literature. Clin Neuropharmacol 36(6):203–215, 2013 24201231

Green AI, Drake RE, Brunette MF, Noordsy DL: Schizophrenia and co-occurring substance use disorder. Am J Psychiatry 164(3):402–408, 2007 17329463

Khantzian EJ: The self-medication hypothesis of substance use disorders: a reconsideration and recent applications. Harv Rev Psychiatry 4(5):231–244, 1997 9385000

Mesholam-Gately RI, Gibson LE, Seidman LJ, et al: Schizophrenia and co-occurring substance use disorder: Reward, olfaction, and clozapine. Schizophr Res 155(1–3):45–51, 2014 24685823

Murthy P, Chand P: Treatment of dual diagnosis disorders. Curr Opin Psychiatry 25(3):194–200, 2012 22395768

Ziedonis DM, Fan X, Bizamcer AN, et al: Co-occurring addiction and psychotic disorders, in The ASAM Principles of Addiction Medicine, 5th Edition. Edited by Ries RK, Fiellin DA, Miller SC, et al. Philadelphia, PA, Lippincott Williams & Wilkins, 2014, pp 1346–1364

# 7

# PERSONALITY DISORDERS

*John W. Barnhill, M.D.*
*Jonathan D. Avery, M.D.*

In this chapter, we discuss the identification and treatment of co-occurring substance use disorders (SUDs) and personality disorders (PDs), with a focus on borderline personality disorder (BPD). While these co-occurring disorders are challenging to treat, it is important to contemporaneously address personality and substance use for two reasons. First, treatment of SUDs requires an alliance, and the alliance will likely be undercut if the clinician does not understand and take into consideration the patient's personality style. Second, people with co-occurring SUDs and PDs often fare poorly in treatment, and there is evidence for the efficacy of simultaneous treatment.

One reason that this effort is challenging is that an individual who uses one substance of abuse can appear wildly different when seen during withdrawal, during acute intoxication, and during persistent abuse. That same patient will look quite different while using a different substance or while using multiple substances. And that same person will think, feel, and behave differently after an extended period of sobriety. Since personality is defined as an enduring pattern of cognition, emotion, motivation, and behavior—and all of these are affected by substances—it can feel difficult to assess and potentially treat personality disorders in people with an active SUD.

An effort to identify a PD—or at least a personality style—is important to the treatment of people with co-occurring SUDs for a variety of reasons. At the least, the clinician's own interviewing style may be more effective if it is adapted to more effectively fit with that of the patient's personality (MacKinnon et al. 2016).

Psychoactive substances can also directly lead to symptom constellations that overlap significantly with the DSM-5 PDs. Antisocial personality disorder (ASPD) is perhaps the most likely to be misdiagnosed in individuals with SUDs, even with the DSM-5 caveat that the diagnosis should be used cautiously in people with SUDs. The reason for this potential misdiagnosis is partly because substances can directly lead people to callous behavior, but also because it is difficult to abuse an expensive and illicit substance without breaking the law and being dishonest.

When a PD is being considered, it is often helpful for the clinician to try to clarify PDs that might have existed prior to the onset of the substance abuse. This is complicated by the fact that substance abuse often starts during adolescence, when personality is still in formation, and by the reality that such data are retrospective and liable to error, even if collateral information is available.

The following case will feature aspects of many of these issues.

---

## Clinical Case

Molly is a 27-year-old woman who presents to an outpatient psychiatric clinic a few days after discharge from a 7-day inpatient psychiatric hospitalization. Molly's initial request was for some sort of treatment to get her life back together.

Molly says she had been admitted to the psychiatric hospital after an overdose in which she took 30 of her own sertraline tablets (1,500 mg), 30 of her own clonazepam tablets (30 mg), and half a liter of vodka. The trigger for the overdose was a cascade of difficult interpersonal events, including quitting her job, "huge fights" with her boyfriend, and financial difficulties that she attributed to being "the grasshopper rather than the ant." When asked to explain what that meant, Molly suggested that the interviewer read more books but clarified that she was not a saver or planner and instead tended to live for the moment. Soon after taking the overdose, she called her mother—who lived in another state—and was in the midst of explaining her many difficulties when she apparently fell asleep. The mother called 911, and Molly was brought to the hospital, where she was immediately intubated and stabilized.

During the acute medical admission, Molly was found to have a blood alcohol level of 352, an MCV of 102, an AST/ALT of 65/32, and a toxicology screen positive for cocaine.

After 5 days of stabilization, which included no signs or symptoms of alcohol withdrawal, Molly was transferred to a nearby psychiatric unit for evaluation of suicidality. That psychiatric hospitalization focused on developing an alliance, a safety assessment, and accumulation of collateral information. After reviewing out-of-town medical charts and from meetings with Molly, Molly's boyfriend, and her parents (who had flown in for sessions), it appeared that Molly's recent behavior was not new. She had been abusing alcohol and cocaine since she was in college, which had led to numerous difficulties with friends and with the law. She had been arrested twice for shoplifting and three times for driving under the influence (DUI). After losing her driver's license, she convinced her boyfriend to move with her to New York so that she wouldn't need a car. There was a general agreement that there was a "Good Molly," who was terrific, and a "Bad Molly," who was scary. The good Molly was engagingly funny, thrived in school, had a wide array of "awesome" friends, and was succeeding in a highly competitive, creative field. The bad Molly abused whatever drugs she could find, cheated on boyfriends, stole from family and friends, "freaked out" whenever things did not go her way, and tended to get desperately and inconsolably needy—especially when drunk and high.

Her parents said that Molly had been a fun and precocious child but had become difficult the "minute she exploded into puberty." It was at that point that her beloved older brother started calling her by new nicknames: "Jekyll" and "Hyde."

Molly's parents were visibly distraught while discussing her failed treatments. She had tried three inpatient drug rehabilitation centers, three different kinds of 12-step programs (Alcoholics Anonymous, Cocaine Anonymous, and Smart Recovery), and an outpatient drug program that featured groups and individual counseling. She had seen three different psychiatrists. One had diagnosed her with only the cocaine and alcohol use disorders, while the other two psychiatrists had diagnosed her with atypical bipolar disorder. Molly had tried multiple medications, including lithium and valproic acid. While these medications reached therapeutic levels for several months each, the primary effects of both were weight gain and cognitive slowing, neither of which had been acceptable to Molly. In addition, Molly had tried diazepam and clonazepam, which she says made her worse rather than better, as well as two different antidepressants, which she said "did nothing," though she thought one of them might have worsened her insomnia.

At the time of the initial presentation, Molly is an attractive young woman who is lively and engaging. She is composed and articulate. Although "things had gotten out of hand," she is "back to baseline" and unsure if she really needs treatment. She denies having been suicidal for one moment since her overdose. She says she had made two prior overdoses that she had slept off without telling anyone, which she seemed to be using to reassure the interviewer that she could take care of herself.

In regard to her history, Molly says that her moods were like clockwork: they went back and forth like a metronome and then she would occasionally go "cuckoo." When asked what that meant, she said she either felt "fine and normal" or felt terrible, which meant "alone, paranoid, furious, self-loathing, manicky, the usual cluster of horrors." When feeling terrible, she sometimes cut herself—when the interviewer asked, she showed a pattern of dozens of thin, healed scars on her upper left arm and on both upper thighs. These cuts were secrets known only to boyfriends and were used to privately help regulate her mood. Drugs also helped control her mood. Cocaine worked best since it was "great at shaking up the moody doldrums," and it also helped her get "crazy social," which meant she could go to any party or bar and "never leave alone." She felt guilty about this recurrent behavior, though she almost invariably attributed this behavior to a boyfriend's negligence or inattentiveness.

Molly's early history was notable for teenage recklessness, particularly in regard to dating older boys and men. She had been able to maintain excellent grades during high school, which she attributed to her avoidance of all drugs and alcohol until college, though she added that she "quickly made up for lost time." Molly and her mother agree that they were extremely close. Molly smilingly adds that her mother probably thought it was "less a symbiotic relationship than a parasitic one," while her mother responds that she loves her daughter and didn't mind the hourly texts but that it did get frustrating when her daughter wanted help to make the tiniest decisions but would invariably argue with the suggestions. Molly and her family are very interested in a treatment recommendation that might arrest her "spiral of misery."

# Discussion

Before a treatment recommendation can be made, Molly needs an accurate diagnosis. Treating substance use disorders alone has been unsuccessful. Treating Molly's dysphoria with antidepressant medications has failed. Diagnosing her lability as atypical bipolar disorder led to unsuccessful trials of mood stabilizers. What else should be considered and addressed?

Among multiple possible diagnoses, borderline personality disorder (BPD) appears most likely. Her substance abuse may fuel her lability, but Molly seems to have developed core BPD symptomatology during an adolescence in which she seems not to have abused substances. In particular, Molly has demonstrated a pervasive pattern of interpersonal instability that includes vulnerability to abandonment; splitting (with extremes of idealization and devaluation); an unstable sense of self (Jekyll and Hyde); recurrent suicidality and self-injurious behavior (the cutting); affective instability; a sense of emptiness; and symptoms of excess anger and paranoia. Her symptoms easily meet DSM-5 criteria for BPD. The co-occurrence of BPD and SUDs is common (Tomko et al. 2014), with rates of BPD as high as 65% among patients with SUDs (Trull et al. 2000). Further, this particular co-occurrence has been associated with a worse functional outcome and increased rates of self-harm and suicidal behavior (Gunderson 2008; Lee et al. 2015; McMain and Ellery 2008).

A BPD diagnosis can be missed for multiple reasons, including the reality that many psychiatrists do not feel equipped to treat BPD. Nevertheless, as is true for most people with co-occurring disorders, Molly's "spiral of misery" is unlikely to be slowed unless the clinician addresses all of her disorders rather than just the one that seems most easily treated by that particular clinician. Treatment of co-occurring BPD and SUDs is addressed in the next section.

In addition to BPD, it would be important to look specifically for posttraumatic stress disorder (PTSD). Multiple bits of information point to possible PTSD. Molly makes it clear that she has been recklessly engaging in sexual relationships while intoxicated, which greatly increases the likelihood of a traumatic event (or suggests that she may be engaging in re-enactments of earlier trauma). She gets distraught and self-loathing, but what is that about? Does she have intrusive memories that fuel some of her substance abuse? Does she avoid memories or experiences that she finds traumatic? We know that she has frequently negative mood states, but might recollections of a traumatic experience trigger them? Might some of her hyperarousal and excess reactivity be related to a traumatic event? Of course, we do not know if Molly experienced a trauma (or multiple traumas), much less if she has symptoms related to the trauma, but it is unlikely that the interviewer will uncover such a history without tactful but persistent exploration.

In addition to the apparent cocaine and alcohol use disorders, it would not be surprising if she had other SUDs. It would be useful to ask about specific substances of abuse, and such a tactful exploration might need to be repeated several times over the course of weeks or months in order to get a complete story. From a medical perspective, it would be useful to check for HIV and hepatitis C. Although Molly denies intravenous substance use, she is at risk for both of these infections, and she is also at risk for forgetting or avoiding some of her own history. HIV is particularly implicated in triggering manic-like behavior, even in patients who have yet to be diagnosed with HIV/AIDS.

Previous psychiatrists appear to have diagnosed her with mood disorders, particularly atypical bipolar disorder and perhaps depression. Their diagnoses do fit some of her symptoms, particularly her apparently cyclical dysphoria and "manicky" behavior. The case does not clarify the relationship between the substance use and these psychiatric symptoms, and so it would be difficult to have confidence in whether Molly might have a bipolar spectrum disorder or whether these symptoms are substance induced. Clarification would be important, especially since, even if we are confident that she has BPD, it is also true that 20% of people with BPD also have bipolar disorder.

Molly has a history of DUIs, shoplifting from stores, and stealing from friends and family. These might indicate that she has ASPD, but, as described in the introduction, these behaviors might be more accurately described as drug-related behavior. It would be helpful to explore these behaviors more fully with Molly, and to get a better understanding of her personality prior to the drug use. However, it is likely that she stole for the money to buy cocaine and that her DUIs were attributable to the simple reality that she was frequently impaired and impulsive rather than willfully putting other people at risk. In the unlikely event that Molly does have ASPD, her prognosis for therapy becomes more guarded, and her treatment might need to be further adapted. There is the most evidence for treatment of BPD and SUDs, which will be discussed below, and little evidence for effective treatments of the other PDs, especially when they are co-occurring with SUDs.

## Treatment

Treatment plans are a negotiation. An important phase of the negotiation is for the clinician to present an understanding of the situation, followed by the patient having a chance to participate in the development of both the diagnosis and treatment plan. Molly is not a child, but she may prefer to have her parents present for at least part of this discussion. In this particular case, if the clinician intends to present a diagnosis of BPD with the SUDs, the patient and her family may well be relieved to be able to put a name to a cluster of behaviors that might otherwise not make sense.

A broad biopsychosocial approach is at the core of the treatment for co-occurring BPD and SUDs. Without an integrated treatment plan, Molly's problems are likely to persist, and even if she avoids suicide, she will continue to fall off the normal trajectory of young adulthood.

## PSYCHOTHERAPEUTIC AND PSYCHOSOCIAL INTERVENTIONS

Psychotherapy is generally considered the first-line treatment for patients with BPD, with or without a co-occurring SUD. *Dialectical behavior therapy* (DBT) has the most evidence for efficacy. This therapy involves individual and group modalities that combine standard cognitive-behavioral approaches with mindfulness, distress tolerance, and acceptance. Both regularly practiced DBT and modified DBT treatments that also explicitly address substance use have been shown to be helpful (Lee et al. 2015; Linehan et al. 2002). DBT groups are now a component of most substance use treatment facilities.

Other psychotherapies for BPD, including psychodynamic psychotherapy, cognitive-behavioral therapy (CBT), and schema therapy, have been studied using evidence-based manuals. For people with co-occurring BPD and SUDs, two of the best-studied therapies are *dynamic deconstructive psychotherapy* (DDP) and *dual-focused schema therapy* (DFST) (Lee et al. 2015). DDP is a modified and manualized weekly psychodynamic psychotherapy. It has been shown, like DBT, to decrease suicidal behavior and other core symptoms of BPD, as well as substance use (Gregory et al. 2010). DFST works on maladaptive schemas, such as negative beliefs about oneself, coping skills, and relapse prevention (Lee et al. 2015).

There are limited data on the effectiveness of 12-step groups or other peer-led interventions for individuals with BPD and SUDs. There is concern, at times, that an individual with BPD may disrupt the 12-step group. At the same time, such groups may help individuals with BPD find a crucial sense of community and meaning.

## PHARMACOLOGICAL INTERVENTIONS

Patients with BPD often end up taking many medications targeted at their different symptoms. There are limited data, however, that these phar-

macological interventions can help with the emptiness, identity disturbance, and abandonment that form the core symptoms of BPD (Stoffers
et al. 2010). Affective or impulsive symptoms may improve with second-generation antipsychotics, mood stabilizers, and dietary supple-
mentation with omega-3 fatty acids, but these gains tend to be modest
(Stoffers et al. 2010). Among these medications, topiramate is increasingly being used in the treatment of individuals with BPD and SUDs, because it has been shown to help in the treatment of both conditions (Litten et al. 2016). Benzodiazepines, while frequently prescribed for BPD,
can lead to addiction and, as seems to be the case with Molly, may actually be disinhibiting rather than calming (Saïas and Gallarda 2008).

It may be useful to pharmacologically target Molly's mood instability
with a medication like topiramate. She did not appear to get a positive effect from previous trials of valproic acid and lithium, but she also did
not take these medications as part of an integrated treatment plan. Even
more evidence exists for the usefulness of medications that have been
shown to be effective for the SUDs, and so it would certainly be reasonable to consider the use of naltrexone or disulfiram for Molly's alcohol use
disorder.

All of the above recommendations would need to be discussed with
the patient, since, at the very least, she is the one who would need to
go forward with this treatment plan. Although it might seem simpler
to focus on one aspect of her problem (e.g., choosing the alcohol or the
cocaine or the depression or the mood instability or the personality disorder), Molly's optimal chance for a recovery and a return to a normal
young adulthood is an integrated, evidence-based approach to her
disorders.

## KEY POINTS

- Psychoactive substances can also directly lead to symptom
  constellations that overlap significantly with the DSM-5 personality disorders.

- The co-occurrence of borderline personality disorder (BPD)
  and substance use disorders (SUDs) is common, with rates of
  BPD as high as 65% among patients with SUDs.

- Psychotherapy is generally considered the first-line treatment
  for patients with BPD, with or without a co-occurring SUD.

# Questions

1. Which of the following may make it difficult to diagnosis a personality disorder in an individual who is misusing substances?

   A. Few periods of abstinence.
   B. Late onset of substance use.
   C. Strong support system.
   D. Reliable historian.

2. Which of the following treatments has the most evidence for efficacy in individuals with borderline personality disorder (BPD) and substance use disorders?

   A. Medication management.
   B. Dialectical behavior therapy (DBT).
   C. Psychodynamic psychotherapy.
   D. 12-step groups.

3. Which of the following medications should be avoided or used with caution in an individual with BPD and a substance use disorder?

   A. Naltrexone.
   B. Lamotrigine.
   C. Lorazepam.
   D. Topiramate.

# References

Gregory RJ, DeLucia-Deranja E, Mogle JA: Dynamic deconstructive psychotherapy versus optimized community care for borderline personality disorder co-occurring with alcohol use disorders: a 30-month follow-up. J Nerv Ment Dis 198(4):292–298, 2010 20386259

Gunderson JG: Borderline Personality Disorder: A Clinical Guide, 2nd Edition. Washington, DC, American Psychiatric Publishing, 2008

Lee NK, Cameron J, Jenner L: A systematic review of interventions for co-occurring substance use and borderline personality disorders. Drug Alcohol Rev 34(6):663–672, 2015 25919396

Linehan MM, Dimeff LA, Reynolds SK, et al: Dialectical behavior therapy versus comprehensive validation therapy plus 12-step for the treatment of opioid dependent women meeting criteria for borderline personality disorder. Drug Alcohol Depend 67(1):13–26, 2002 12062776

Litten RZ, Wilford BB, Falk DE, et al: Potential medications for the treatment of alcohol use disorder: An evaluation of clinical efficacy and safety. Subst Abus 37(2):286–298, 2016 26928397

MacKinnon RA, Michels R, Buckley PJ: The Psychiatric Interview in Clinical Practice, 3rd Edition. Arlington, VA, American Psychiatric Association Publishing, 2016

McMain S, Ellery M: Screening and assessment of personality disorders in addiction treatment settings. Int J Ment Health Addict 6:20–31, 2008

Saïas T, Gallarda T: [Paradoxical aggressive reactions to benzodiazepine use: a review]. Encephale 34(4):330–336, 2008 18922233

Stoffers J, Völlm BA, Rücker G, et al: Pharmacological interventions for borderline personality disorder. Cochrane Database Syst Rev (6):CD005653, 2010 20556762

Tomko RL, Trull TJ, Wood PK, Sher KJ: Characteristics of borderline personality disorder in a community sample: comorbidity, treatment utilization, and general functioning. J Pers Disord 28(5):734–750, 2014 25248122

Trull TJ, Sher KJ, Minks-Brown C, et al: Borderline personality disorder and substance use disorders: a review and integration. Clin Psychol Rev 20(2):235–253, 2000 10721499

# ATTENTION-DEFICIT/ HYPERACTIVITY DISORDER

*Sean X. Luo, M.D., Ph.D.*

*Frances R. Levin, M.D.*

Substance use disorders (SUDs) tend to co-occur with attention-deficit/ hyperactivity disorder (ADHD) (Kessler et al. 2006; Mariani and Levin 2007; van Emmerik-van Oortmerssen et al. 2012; Wilens 2004; Wilens et al. 1998). The use of psychoactive substances can also be directly impli- cated in a variety of types of executive dysfunction that may or not be part of ADHD. These dysfunctions can include cardinal symptoms of ADHD, such as inattention (e.g., careless mistakes, daydreaming, dis- organization) and hyperactivity (e.g., fidgeting, impatience, nonstop talking) (Brown et al. 2001). In this chapter, we present a clinical case and then discuss an evidence-based approach to understanding and treating patients who present with what can be a bewildering assort- ment of symptoms.

## Clinical Case

Richard is a 32-year-old, single man who has episodically worked part time as a computer programmer but who has been unemployed much of the time since dropping out of college a decade earlier. He was referred for a psychiatric evaluation after his parents had become increasingly frustrated by his behavior, threatening to "kick him out" of their house if he didn't "get sober, get a job, and get a life."

The patient reports he "has been a mess" his whole life, with a persistent inability to function effectively at work, at school, and with friends. He has dated "a little" but the relationships "fizzle out" within weeks or months. He believes his biggest problem is his cocaine use. Richard describes an intensifying use in the 6 months since he was most recently fired. He describes spending $200–$300 (about 1–3 grams) every weekend in a binge pattern with his friends. He reports significant withdrawal symptoms after a weekend binge, including insomnia, daytime sleepiness, depressive mood, poor concentration, and food binges. He has long had sleep-wake reversals, but he describes an intensifying pattern in which he would sleep most of the day and play video games at night. Since he has never moved away from home, this behavior was quite noticeable and worrisome to his parents, who insisted he seek treatment.

Richard reports a chronic history of inattention, impulsivity, and procrastination. He was diagnosed with ADHD in seventh grade. A several-month trial of immediate-release methylphenidate at that time led to significant clinical improvement (according to his mother) and to significant side effects (according to Richard). He specifically denies recalling any behavioral improvement on the methylphenidate, adding that all he recalls was "feeling jittery" and "tunnel vision."

Richard began to smoke marijuana during high school, increasing to daily use during college. He quit cannabis 2 years earlier and now only smokes occasionally. He also drinks alcohol socially, but "not like at college," when he would have 10–15 drinks on weekends and 2–5 drinks every night during the week. He experimented with oral opioids such as OxyContin but never sustained a regular pattern of use. He describes some other "random experimentation" during college, including LSD, mushrooms, and crystal methamphetamine, but denies having used any other drugs in over 10 years. In his view, his only "problem drug" is the cocaine. He believes the cocaine hurt his motivation and ability to sustain school and work, but he also feels ambivalent about cutting down or staying abstinent, stating "nothing in my life is as good as cocaine."

In regard to a more detailed social history, Richard is an only child born to middle-class parents. He and his parents agree that he graduated from high school with mediocre grades and poor attendance. He attended several semesters at a local community college before dropping out. While he had a knack for computer science, he was often unable to concentrate and complete assignments even in subjects that he found interesting. He has worked part time as a computer programmer but has spent most of the last decade playing video games in his parents' basement.

---

# Discussion

Richard has a serious history of substance misuse, which no doubt impacts on his ability to function. At the same time, he was diagnosed with ADHD prior to using illicit substances. While the SUDs and the ADHD seem to co-occur, which is a common scenario, it is also common for evaluating clinicians to recognize the externalizing behaviors and relatively "loud" problems associated with substance use and not recognize ADHD and its powerful effect on the lives of young people like Richard. While Richard's ADHD diagnosis appears fairly clear, it is less clear for other people. For example, it becomes difficult to assess symptoms related to attention and hyperactivity if they develop while an early adolescent is in the early phase of a SUD or if the ADHD symptoms are not initially well documented. In such cases, it can be helpful to assess ADHD symptoms after a period of time away from substances of abuse. In practice, however, a month or two of abstinence can be difficult to achieve without first managing the patient's ADHD symptoms.

Ideally, ADHD and SUDs would be evaluated and treated simultaneously, and within the context of a comprehensive overall evaluation of the patient. In Richard's case, the clinical story should not just focus on the ADHD and SUD but include details of his strengths as well as his impairments.

Although the diagnosis of ADHD is primarily clinical, a variety of rating scales have been developed to assess for ADHD symptoms in adults and adolescents with SUDs. Rating scales are useful not only for screening but also for tracking current symptoms and assessing for treatment response. The 18-item core symptoms from DSM-5 have been shown to be valid and reliable: individuals with these core symptoms also have other objective characteristics of ADHD, such as a typical pattern of comorbidity, genetic associations, and functional neuroimaging features. A summary of some commonly used available diagnostic instruments is included in Table 8–1. Some of the instruments, such as the Adult ADHD Self-Report Scale, Version 1.1, can be administered in as little as 5 minutes to provide a brief, validated assessment of current or past symptom severity (Kessler et al. 2007). A definitive diagnosis of ADHD can be made using a semi-structured psychiatric diagnostic interview such as Conners' Adult ADHD Diagnostic Interview for DSM-IV or the Diagnostic Interview for ADHD in Adults 2.0 (DIVA 2.0), and in clinical practice semi-structured interviews can be modified depending on availability of resources and training.

Blood alcohol levels and urine drug screens should generally be obtained for new patients. Frequent follow-up testing can be useful diagnostically. In addition, some patients are able to delay or discontinue substance use if they know they are soon to get tested. Just as objective toxicology data can help clarify ambiguity, collateral information from the patient's family, friends, and coworkers—if permitted—can be invaluable in trying to clarify history. Other components of the initial evaluation, such as prior psychiatric and family history and social and occupational history, are also useful in determining optimal treatment and considering disposition options.

A thorough evaluation of general medical conditions is very important for co-occurring ADHD and SUDs. Thyroid and cortisol-related conditions (including steroid treatment), and acute metabolic disturbances (including hypoxia, hypercarbia, hypoglycemia, and water and salt imbalance) either due to a general medical condition, effects of psychotropic medications, or substances of abuse, can mimic symptoms of ADHD. Unlike general medical conditions, ADHD usually has a prominent childhood onset. Primary psychiatric disorders such as mood and anxiety disorders are frequently comorbid in this population, and personality disorders are also very common. In this particular case, the patient denied symptoms of primary psychiatric disorders. However, patient self-reports are often inaccurate and contradictory, and collateral information can be very helpful in making a diagnosis.

While SUD and ADHD both warrant simultaneous attention during the evaluation phase, the initial active treatment is usually focused on the SUDs (Riggs 1998). While the comprehensive evaluation of SUDs is beyond the scope of this chapter, the American Society of Addiction Medicine (ASAM) criteria for assessing severity and placement for SUD treatment constitute an evidence-based, well-validated process, and the cri-

**TABLE 8–1.** Commonly used diagnostic scales and interviews for attention-deficit/hyperactivity disorder (ADHD)

| Scale or interview | Administration type | Source |
|---|---|---|
| **Structured instruments for assessing ADHD symptoms** | | |
| Conners' Adult ADHD Diagnostic Interview for DSM-IV | Clinician administered | Epstein J, Johnson DE, Conners CK, Multi-Health Systems, Inc.; http://www.mhs.com |
| Barkley Current Symptoms Scale—Self-Report Form[a] | Self-report | Barkley RA, Murphy KR: *Attention-Deficit Hyperactivity Disorder: A Clinical Workbook*, 2nd Edition. New York, Guilford, 2006 |
| Adult ADHD Self-Report Scale, Version 1.1 (ASRS v1.1) Symptom Checklist | Self-report | World Health Organization; https://add.org/wp-content/uploads/2015/03/adhd-questionnaire-ASRS111.pdf |
| Brown ADD Scales (Brown ADD Rating Scales and Diagnostic Forms) | Clinician administered | Pearson; http://www.pearsonclinical.com |
| Kiddie Schedule for Affective Disorders and Schizophrenia—Present, Lifetime (K-SADS PL) | Clinician administered | http://www.pediatricbipolar.pitt.edu/content.asp?id=2333 |
| **Semi-structured diagnostic interviews** | | |
| Diagnostic Interview for ADHD in Adults, Version 2.0 (DIVA 2.0) | — | DIVA Foundation; http://www.divacenter.eu/ |
| Conners' Adult ADHD Diagnostic Interview for DSM-IV | — | Multi-Health Systems, Inc.; http://www.mhs.com |

[a]Part of the Barkley Adult ADHD Rating Scale–4.

teria can usually be applied in evaluating patients with comorbid ADHD and SUD (Stallvik and Nordahl 2014). The ASAM criteria use a multi-factorial dimensional model, and each patient is evaluated via six separate dimensions (i.e., acute intoxication/withdrawal, physical health, psychological health, readiness to change, tendency to relapse, and living environment). A systematic algorithm allows for the appropriate choice of treatment context (e.g., inpatient vs. outpatient). Treatment planning can be tailored depending on the patient's readiness to change and the potential for relapse and further functional deterioration.

There are a number of theories that try to explain the high rate of co-morbidity between ADHD and SUD. The shared diathesis model stipulates that there is common underlying neurobiology. For example, multiple genetic polymorphisms are associated with both ADHD and SUD (Carpentier et al. 2013). It has also been conjectured that common environmental stressors (e.g., poor interpersonal performance and school failure) and common psychological traits (e.g., impulsivity and conduct problems) contribute to the development of both ADHD and SUD (Molina and Pelham 2014). Standard psychological testing batteries have so far been unable to identify children who go on to develop a SUD, though more subtle evaluation of reward-motivation processes may eventually allow us to make more accurate predictions (Molina and Pelham 2014).

An alternative theory is the self-medication hypothesis: substances are abused to "treat" common ADHD symptoms such as inattention and irritability. This idea is supported by the idea that patients with ADHD exhibit underlying neurocircuitry/neurotransmitter abnormalities, most prominently in dopamine neurotransmission in the limbic striatum (Koob and Volkow 2010). Substances of abuse that have a prominent dopaminergic effect, such as cocaine, can often temporarily alleviate ADHD symptoms. The patient describes the effect of cocaine as "calming" and the only thing that helps him or her feel "happy and normal," which is a common if seemingly paradoxical description of cocaine's effects. These positive effects of cocaine are short lived, however, and the deficit of dopamine release after cocaine use can worsen ADHD symptoms and cause further deterioration, as seen in this patient.

ADHD is underdiagnosed and undertreated in individuals with SUDs. One problem is that the diagnosis is often delayed because of uncertain symptom attribution. For example, is the amotivation or inattention related to ADHD or the substance abuse, or to some combination? A second problem relates to the reality that the primary treatment for ADHD is a psychostimulant, which leads many clinicians to forgo an ADHD diagnosis in order to avoid prescribing a potentially addictive medication to someone with a potentially high risk for abuse.

However, risk of developing a substance use disorder for prescription stimulants, especially the newer, longer-acting formulations, is low, even in patients with comorbid SUDs. The disorganization intrinsic to the lives of patients with untreated ADHD can interfere significantly with employment, school, and relationships, but it can also negatively impact psychotherapy and the treatment for the SUD; if patients forget their appointments and their therapy "homework," they will often be unable to progress with treatment for any of their co-occurring disorders. Addressing ADHD symptoms when SUDs become stabilized is therefore a major focus of clinical attention.

# Treatment

Optimal management of patients with both SUD and ADHD requires a combination of psychotherapeutic and psychosocial interventions and pharmacological interventions. Although treatment of ADHD generally follows stabilization of SUD symptoms, treatment planning is primarily based on access to a variety of treatment modalities, clinical judgment, patient preference, and flexibility and adaptability of both the clinician and the patient.

## PSYCHOTHERAPEUTIC AND PSYCHOSOCIAL INTERVENTIONS

Several psychotherapy modalities have been tested, often in conjunction with pharmacotherapy, in the treatment of ADHD or SUD, but few have been designed to treat both simultaneously. Cognitive-behavioral therapy (CBT) appears to be efficacious for both ADHD (Safren et al. 2010) and SUD (Dutra et al. 2008). CBT for ADHD primarily targets problems with executive functioning: problems with time estimation, initiation of tasks, completion of tasks, changing focus, and organization. New skills are emphasized, including learning to explicitly categorize, prioritize, and differentially motivate for different tasks. Traditional CBT can also be used to address demoralization, anxiety, and perfectionism. Patients often benefit from interventions that are concrete and that focus on specific tasks, such as writing a paper or completing a set of work-related projects in a specific timeframe.

Psychosocial interventions for SUDs generally take a different tack and may start with motivational enhancement therapy (MET), especially when the patient's attitude toward drug use is ambivalent. When the patient's goals for treatment have been established, CBT can then be used to manage emerging symptoms such as craving and impulsive behavior for using and obtaining drugs, as well as establishing better social boundaries. There is also a significant role in using contingency regard ("contingency management") as part of the treatment.

We recommend an integrated approach for psychotherapy for patients with ADHD and SUD. A sample therapeutic plan (adapted as a shorter form of a published protocol) is shown in Table 8–2A (van Emmerik-van Oortmerssen et al. 2013). This shorter version emphasizes flexibility and is tailored to the patient's goals and the symptom severity. Involvement of family and other social support, such as groups and sober companions, is also helpful.

## PHARMACOLOGICAL INTERVENTIONS

Medications have an important role in ADHD treatment. A variety of medications (Table 8–2B) are effective for reducing ADHD symptoms, including stimulants, α-adrenergic agonists, noradrenergic agents, and catecholaminergic antidepressants. Evidence for using psychostimulants in co-occurring ADHD and SUDs is complex and nuanced; clarifying how and when different types of medications are most effective continues to be an active area of research. For example, while some studies using stimulants in cocaine users have shown a general improvement in co-occurring ADHD symptoms (Levin et al. 2007), improvement of cocaine use outcome only occurred when mixed-amphetamine salts were used at robust dosing schedules and in combination with CBT (Levin et al. 2015). Similarly, while methylphenidate improves ADHD symptoms in adults (Winhusen et al. 2010) and adolescents (Riggs et al. 2011), its beneficial effects do not become apparent until baseline severity (Nunes et al. 2013) and other covariates (Tamm et al. 2013) are taken into account. Predictive models that integrate patient characteristics to tailor treatment may represent a novel approach in this area (Luo et al. 2015).

Clinically, we recommend using either atomoxetine or stimulants as a first-line treatment for co-occurring ADHD and SUD. Atomoxetine is particularly helpful for abstinent alcohol-dependent individuals and those whose tic disorders may be worsened by exposure to stimulants— some individuals with tic disorders may have variable changes of their tic symptoms when exposed to a stimulant (Cohen et al. 2015; Cooke and So 2016).

Although they do carry abuse potential, stimulants are more effective than atomoxetine for core ADHD symptoms, and so we do use them in some patients with co-occurring ADHD and SUDs after addressing a number of safety considerations. First, stimulants increase pulse and blood

**TABLE 8–2.** Psychotherapy and medication treatment of comorbid attention-deficit/hyperactivity disorder (ADHD) with substance use disorders (SUDs)

**A. Sample integrated cognitive-behavioral therapy (CBT) treatment plan for comorbid ADHD and SUDs[a]**

| | SUD | ADHD |
|---|---|---|
| Session 1 | Motivational enhancement, clarification of goals | Foundation of executive function |
| Session 2 | Tracking craving, drug use behavior | Tracking symptoms; time management |
| Sessions 3–5 | Core SUD CBT | |
| Sessions 5–8 | Core SUD CBT | Time management; executive functioning |
| Sessions 8–12 | Integrated concepts: decisional analysis, adaptive thinking, consolidation of new skills | |

**B. Pharmacotherapy for ADHD and SUDs**

| Atomoxetine | Nonstimulant | | Noncontrolled |
|---|---|---|---|
| Methylphenidate | Stimulant | Shorter- and longer-acting formulations | Monitor for misuse/diversion |
| Amphetamine | Stimulant | Shorter- and longer-acting formulations | Monitor for misuse/diversion |
| Bupropion | Non–FDA approved | | Also useful for smoking cessation |
| Guanfacine | Non–FDA approved | | |
| Modafanil | Non–FDA approved | | |
| TCA | Non–FDA approved | | |

[a] Adapted from Winhusen et al. 2010 in a shorter form. TCA=tricyclic antidepressant.

pressure, potentially additive to cardiovascular effects of some substances of abuse, like cocaine. Risks of adverse cardiovascular events must be carefully evaluated, and blood pressure should be longitudinally measured. Stimulants may also cause mood lability, anxiety, and agitation, as we see in the case of Richard, who reports that his seventh-grade trial of amphetamines was discontinued because he felt "jittery."

Misuse and diversion are inherent risks for stimulants, though existing data have shown that treatment using stimulants has not yielded a particularly high rate of abuse or diversion. Red flags for misuse or diversion include intoxication or heavier use, demands for a fast-acting and higher-dosing formulation, repeated lost prescriptions, discordant pill count, and multiple prescribers. Appropriate use of stimulants requires vigilant monitoring to ensure that the risk of misuse is mitigated while patients are not under-treated.

# Conclusion

ADHD and SUDs commonly occur together. These conditions may have common underlying biological and environmental causes. Evaluation for and recognition of ADHD and SUDs should occur simultaneously, though active treatment is often initially directed at the SUDs. As is generally the case with patients with SUDs, clinicians should tailor the treatment plan to patient motivation, with the ultimate goal of working with the patient to optimize happiness and social and occupational functioning.

## KEY POINTS

- Substance use disorders (SUDs) tend to co-occur with attention-deficit/hyperactivity disorder (ADHD).

- Optimal management of ADHD can often improve treatment of SUDs, including preventing relapse and reestablishing better psychosocial support and occupational functioning.

- Studies of pharmacological treatment of ADHD indicate that psychostimulants are safe and effective in treating ADHD in patients with SUDs, and diversion and misuse are infrequent if treatment is carefully monitored.

# Questions

1. A patient presents to you for treatment for cocaine use disorder. You conduct a structured interview, which confirms your suspicion of a diagnosis of attention-deficit/hyperactivity disorder (ADHD). Which of the following would be inaccurate in providing psychoeducation for the patient?

    A. "ADHD is very common in patients with substance use disorders. It's possible that part of why it's so difficult for you to quit on your own is because your ADHD symptoms are poorly managed."
    B. "Depression and anxiety are very uncommon symptoms when someone also has ADHD."
    C. "Patients with ADHD are sometimes not diagnosed during childhood, and some ADHD symptoms persist into adulthood."
    D. "Patients who use cocaine have similar rates of ADHD compared to individuals dependent on other drugs."

2. You initiate a trial of psychostimulant for an adolescent patient with comorbid ADHD and SUD. Her parents, however, have significant concerns that she might "get addicted" to the stimulant and sell the stimulant to her friends. Which of the following is incorrect and should not be included as part of your counseling for the family?

    A. "While psychostimulants carry a small risk of abuse, adequate treatment of ADHD is an important factor in successful control of the patient's substance use disorder."
    B. "While diversion is a concern for stimulants, especially in the college-age population, most college students who report using stimulants do so to study for exams or complete papers, rather than to get high."
    C. "While misuse of methylphenidate-based medications has been stable, misuse of prescription amphetamines has been dramatically increasing."
    D. "Longer-acting formulations of psychostimulant generally have a lower liability for misuse compared with immediate-release formulations."

3. Your patient, who has both an alcohol use disorder and a cocaine use disorder, received initial treatment with a long-acting methylphenidate preparation for his ADHD. His symptoms of ADHD

improved but did not fully remit, and he continues to use cocaine sporadically, though he has stopped drinking. Which of the following is *true* for revising his treatment plan?

A. Higher-than-standard dosing of mixed-amphetamine salts may reduce both ADHD and substance use.
B. Atomoxetine is generally ineffective for treating ADHD symptoms in adults with alcohol use disorder.
C. Amphetamines, as opposed to methylphenidate, have been found to increase cocaine use in patients with both alcohol and cocaine use disorders, and are therefore contraindicated in this patient.
D. Cognitive-behavioral therapy (CBT) produces a minimal reduction in ADHD symptoms.

# References

Brown RT, Freeman WS, Perrin JM, et al: Prevalence and assessment of attention-deficit/hyperactivity disorder in primary care settings. Pediatrics 107(3):E43, 2001 11230624

Carpentier PJ, Arias Vasquez A, Hoogman M, et al: Shared and unique genetic contributions to attention deficit/hyperactivity disorder and substance use disorders: a pilot study of six candidate genes. Eur Neuropsychopharmacol 23(6):448–457, 2013 22841130

Cooke T, So TY: Attention deficit hyperactive disorder and occurrence of tic disorders in children and adolescents—what is the verdict? Curr Pediatr Rev 12(3):230-238, 2016 27470148

Cohen SC, Mulqueen JM, Ferracioli-Oda E, et al: Meta-analysis: risk of tics associated with psychostimulant use in randomized, placebo-controlled trials. J Am Acad Child Adolesc Psychiatry 54(9):728–736, 2015 26299294

Dutra L, Stathopoulou G, Basden SL, et al: A meta-analytic review of psychosocial interventions for substance use disorders. Am J Psychiatry 165(2):179–187, 2008 18198270

Kessler RC, Adler L, Barkley R, et al: The prevalence and correlates of adult ADHD in the United States: results from the National Comorbidity Survey Replication. Am J Psychiatry 163(4):716–723, 2006 16585449

Kessler RC, Adler LA, Gruber MJ, et al: Validity of the World Health Organization Adult ADHD Self-Report Scale (ASRS) Screener in a representative sample of health plan members. Int J Methods Psychiatr Res 16(2):52–65, 2007 17623385

Koob GF, Volkow ND: Neurocircuitry of addiction. Neuropsychopharmacology 35(1):217–238, 2010 19710631

Levin FR, Evans SM, Brooks DJ, et al: Treatment of cocaine dependent treatment seekers with adult ADHD: double-blind comparison of methylphenidate and placebo. Drug Alcohol Depend 87(1):20–29, 2007 16930863

Levin FR, Mariani JJ, Specker S, et al: Extended-release mixed amphetamine salts vs placebo for comorbid adult attention-deficit/hyperactivity disorder and cocaine use disorder: a randomized clinical trial. JAMA Psychiatry 72(6):593–602, 2015 25887096

Luo SX, Covey LS, Hu MC, et al: Toward personalized smoking-cessation treatment: Using a predictive modeling approach to guide decisions regarding stimulant medication treatment of attention-deficit/hyperactivity disorder (ADHD) in smokers. Am J Addict 24(4):348–356, 2015 25659348

Mariani JJ, Levin FR: Treatment strategies for co-occurring ADHD and substance use disorders. Am J Addict 16(Suppl 1):45–54; quiz 55–56, 2007 17453606

Molina BS, Pelham WE Jr: Attention-deficit/hyperactivity disorder and risk of substance use disorder: developmental considerations, potential pathways, and opportunities for research. Annu Rev Clin Psychol 10:607–639, 2014 24437435

Nunes EV, Covey LS, Brigham G, et al: Treating nicotine dependence by targeting attention-deficit/ hyperactivity disorder (ADHD) with OROS methylphenidate: the role of baseline ADHD severity and treatment response. J Clin Psychiatry 74(10):983–990, 2013 24229749

Riggs PD: Clinical approach to treatment of ADHD in adolescents with substance use disorders and conduct disorder. J Am Acad Child Adolesc Psychiatry 37(3):331–332, 1998 9519639

Riggs PD, Winhusen T, Davies RD, et al: Randomized controlled trial of osmotic-release methylphenidate with cognitive-behavioral therapy in adolescents with attention-deficit/hyperactivity disorder and substance use disorders. J Am Acad Child Adolesc Psychiatry 50(9):903–914, 2011 21871372

Safren SA, Sprich S, Mimiaga MJ, et al: Cognitive behavioral therapy vs relaxation with educational support for medication-treated adults with ADHD and persistent symptoms: a randomized controlled trial. JAMA 304(8):875–880, 2010 20736471

Stallvik M, Nordahl HM: Convergent validity of the ASAM criteria in co-occurring disorders. J Dual Diagn 10(2):68–78, 2014 25392248

Tamm L, Trello-Rishel K, Riggs P, et al: Predictors of treatment response in adolescents with comorbid substance use disorder and attention-deficit/hyperactivity disorder. J Subst Abuse Treat 44(2):224–230, 2013 22889694

van Emmerik-van Oortmerssen K, van de Glind G, van den Brink W, et al: Prevalence of attention-deficit hyperactivity disorder in substance use disorder patients: a meta-analysis and meta-regression analysis. Drug Alcohol Depend 122(1-2):11–19, 2012 22209385

van Emmerik-van Oortmerssen K, Vedel E, Koeter MW, et al: Investigating the efficacy of integrated cognitive behavioral therapy for adult treatment seeking substance use disorder patients with comorbid ADHD: study protocol of a randomized controlled trial. BMC Psychiatry 13:132, 2013 23663651

Wilens TE: Attention-deficit/hyperactivity disorder and the substance use disorders: the nature of the relationship, subtypes at risk, and treatment issues. Psychiatr Clin North Am 27(2):283–301, 2004 15063998

Wilens TE, Biederman J, Mick E: Does ADHD affect the course of substance abuse? Findings from a sample of adults with and without ADHD. Am J Addict 7(2):156–163, 1998 9598219

Winhusen TM, Somoza EC, Brigham GS, et al: Impact of attention-deficit/hyperactivity disorder (ADHD) treatment on smoking cessation intervention in ADHD smokers: a randomized, double-blind, placebo-controlled trial. J Clin Psychiatry 71(12):1680–1688, 2010 20492837

# EATING DISORDERS

*Sean P. Kerrigan, M.D.*
*Evelyn Attia, M.D.*

Eating disorders (EDs) and substance use disorders (SUDs) frequently co-occur. At times, the two co-occurring disorders appear to have developed independently, but there is generally some connection. Some individuals who have an ED abuse substances in an effort to control their appetite and/or weight. Other people have developed a SUD in the context of mood instability, dysphoria, or anxiety that may also play a role in their ED. Some people with EDs develop a SUD to manage their feelings of shame and isolation, while for others, social norms, peer pressure, and/or genetics play a deciding role. For many patients with both an ED and SUD, it can be difficult to tease apart which of these issues is particularly crucial or primary.

The National Center on Addiction and Substance Abuse (CASA) at Columbia University (2003) concluded in a landmark 3-year study that individuals with EDs are up to 5 times likelier to abuse alcohol or illicit drugs than peers without these disorders, and that individuals who abuse alcohol or illicit drugs are up to 11 times likelier to have EDs than control populations. Furthermore, up to 50% of individuals with an ED abuse alcohol or illicit drugs compared with approximately 9% in the general population (National Center on Addiction and Substance Abuse at Columbia University 2003).

The following case reflects a fairly typical patient with a co-occurring ED and SUD. The discussion will focus on the assessment and evidence-based treatments.

## Clinical Case

Elena is a 19-year-old woman who was referred for an outpatient psychiatric evaluation by her parents because of an inability to function effectively during her first semester of college. While Elena's parents are concerned about her late nights, missed classes, and poor grades, Elena believes she is just having a "typical" first year of college. According to Elena, her parents are too focused on disordered eating and alcohol abuse.

During her first evaluation session, Elena says that she knows that her parents are concerned about her drinking, especially since it seems to be leading her to being unable to wake up in time for her 9 A.M. classes. She agrees that she sometimes "overdoes it" but explains that most of her drinking is "social" and not a problem. She describes nightly drinking of perhaps 4–6 beers, as well as weekend drinking that starts at noon on Friday. She agrees that she has experienced a few blackouts, but she insists that "blackouts are what you get when you get really drunk." She adds that this behavior sounds bad but isn't dangerous since she and a friend always drink together and watch out for each other. Her main problem with the drinking is that it has led to a 10-pound weight gain. She adds that she knows she probably looks normal to outsiders, but that she thinks about her weight "all the time."

When asked if she is doing anything to control her weight gain, Elena says that she just does "the usual things." For example, she tends not to eat when she knows she is going to be drinking since she knows alcohol has a lot of empty calories and that she can get drunk faster without food. Elena adds that the one downside to drinking is that it often leads her to overeat on junk food, which is freely available on campus, and especially at parties. Sometimes, she says, she gets so hungry that she eats "a massive amount," but that she is generally very serious about her diet. The clinician notices that Elena has scrapes on her knuckles and that her face seems somewhat puffy, so she asks about vomiting. Elena pauses and agrees that she sometimes vomits while drunk and that she has begun to induce vomiting after she eats too much. She insists that she purges only a few times per week and that it is under control. When asked if she also uses laxatives, Elena pauses and says, "Only occasionally."

Elena says her main complaints are fatigue, insomnia, school difficulties, and her parents giving her a hard time. She denies any psychiatric history prior to college. She agrees that she keeps her purging a secret, but she is confident that she will outgrow it. She told her parents she would go to therapy, however, since otherwise her parents would refuse to pay for her sorority and would instead make her live at home.

# Discussion

Elena's story is somewhat typical in that she did not seek treatment on her own and then tries to minimize and normalize the extent of her difficulties with eating and alcohol. While this chapter will focus on these co-occurring disorders, it is important to be aware that we need to know significantly more about this young woman or else her treatment will be incomplete. For example, does she have additional psychiatric diagnoses, such as anxiety or depression? Recognition of these co-occurring disorders might be crucial in progressing in treatment. In addition, has anything traumatic occurred while Elena was intoxicated, and if so, might her reaction to the trauma contribute to further dangerous behavior? Perhaps most crucially, Elena appears to be externally motivated to pursue treatment—if she doesn't attend sessions, her parents will reduce financial support. The best diagnostic formulation and most highly developed treatment plan will be meaningless if Elena refuses to attend further sessions. For these reasons, the initial sessions need to balance the need to obtain historical information with the imperative to develop a working alliance and to help motivate Elena into therapeutic involvement.

From what we understand, Elena has an ED characterized by bingeing, purging, weight preoccupation, attempts to curb her binges, and a social/physical impact that includes fatigue, insomnia, and poor school performance. If we assume that these behaviors meet the minimum DSM-5 criteria of weekly behaviors for 3 months, she appears to have fairly classic bulimia nervosa (BN) (American Psychiatric Association 2013). Other EDs are less likely. If she were at a greatly reduced weight, then she would be more likely to have anorexia nervosa, binge-eating/purging type. If weight preoccupation were not a primary issue, and if she did not purge, Elena might then have binge-eating disorder. If her motivation were related not to weight loss but instead to, for example, abdominal pain, she might have avoidant/restrictive food intake disorder (ARFID). The ED diagnosis would also become more unclear if the clinician viewed her vomiting and disordered eating as secondary to alcohol misuse. In Elena's case, however, it appears that she has BN complicated by the alcohol use.

As is true for the eating issues, Elena minimizes her alcohol use. It can be tempting to agree with patients when they argue that "everyone is doing it." While Elena is not immediately forthcoming, she does appear to be drinking frequently, experiencing blackouts, exposing herself to potentially dangerous situations, and having significant academic consequences. She clearly qualifies for an alcohol use disorder. Although the case presentation does not address the issue, it will be important to clarify possible alcohol withdrawal phenomena, especially given the serious medical consequences if left untreated.

It will be useful to explore Elena's use of alcohol to improve mood, manage anger, and/or help control impulsive eating (Stock et al. 2002). Alcohol use disorders are particularly common in ED subgroups with purging behaviors. They may be associated with emotional dysregulation and impulsivity, at times in the form of binge drinking after failed attempts to restrict calories. For example, it would not be surprising if Elena's attempt to reduce purging would lead to an intensification of her alcohol use. This "see-saw" behavior can lead to a persistent pattern of reactive coping to help regain control over mood and anxiety (American Psychiatric Association 2013).

For many ED patients, substances may also be abused in order to lose weight, and it would be useful to tactfully explore many different substances that Elena might be using. As we see with Elena, over-the-counter laxatives are most common and are used in up to 75% of ED patients (Mitchell et al. 1997). Stimulants are also commonly used, largely because they tend to suppress appetite (American Psychiatric Association 2013). Many people with EDs prefer coffee, diet soda, and exercise supplements, because they have minimal social stigma, widespread availability, no legal risks, and fewer side effects than illicit stimulants such as cocaine or methamphetamine (American Psychiatric Association 2013). Stimulants may also be consumed in excess to treat the fatigue that frequently accompanies ED (American Psychiatric Association 2013). Nicotine is also a stimulant, and cigarettes are abused with significantly greater frequency in ED patients than in healthy individuals (Krug et al. 2008). Several cigarette brands have molded past advertising campaigns for women around an association between "longer and thinner" cigarette lines and a svelte physique, comparing their customers posi-tively to women who choose dessert after meals (American Psychiatric Association 2013; Jeffers et al. 2013). Patients may also resort to pre-scribed medications. For example, thyroid hormone can increase me-tabolism, while exogenous insulin can reduce absorption of calories (Powers 1997). Abuse of many of the above substances can have a vari-ety of negative physiological consequences, including cardiovascular and metabolic problems (Powers 1997). It behooves the clinician to be attentive to possible EDs when patients are found to be abusing any substance that enhances metabolism, decreases appetite, or reduces ab-sorption of food.

It appears that the presence of a preexisting ED increases the likelihood of the development of a SUD more than a SUD increases the likelihood of the development of an ED (Franko et al. 2005). Some have argued that this pattern reflects the widespread effort to lose weight that leads peo-ple to turn to substances such as psychostimulants, which then leads to a secondary SUD (Jeffers et al. 2013). For other patients, the mood insta-bility, impulsivity, and personality issues that are commonly associated with purging may be the crucial factor associated with substance use. For still other patients—particularly women—depression and disgust with body image are risk factors for developing a co-occurring alcohol use disorder (Franko et al. 2005).

As we see with Elena, the highest prevalence of substance use lies with bulimia nervosa and binge-eating disorder. Similarly, patients with signs and symptoms meeting criteria for AN binge-eating/purging type appear to have a significantly higher rate of substance abuse treat-ment by roughly two-thirds compared with their restriction-focused counterparts (Root et al. 2010), suggesting that there may be a stronger correlation between substance misuse and generalized binge-purge symp-toms themselves, rather than between substance misuse and a specific eating disorder diagnosis (Gregorowski et al. 2013).

AN and BN have been conceptualized as "addictive syndromes," in which food (or its absence) is the substance of choice. It seems more likely, however, that the confluence of environmental, genetic, psycho-logical, and neurobiological factors that lead to the development of an ED is qualitatively different than the addictions, which appear more clearly to reflect problems with dopamine-driven reward pathways. The genesis of AN in particular shares more common ground with anxiety-spectrum diagnoses such as obsessive-compulsive disorder, in which compulsive food strategies are repeatedly used to alleviate (or distract from) obsessive worries about one's body shape (Barbarich-Marsteller et al. 2011).

# Treatment

As is generally true, treatment begins during the assessment, and it is crucial to promote an alliance during the initial information gathering. In addition, although it may be useful to explore historical details into Elena's ED and alcohol use disorder, an "origin-agnostic" approach is generally recommended at the onset of treatment. The causes of both disorders are typically multifactorial, for example, and the assumption or delegation of blame can complicate recovery from these co-occurring disorders. In Elena's case, historical details need to be explored tactfully, especially since she doesn't appear to believe that she has clinically relevant problems.

Given these limitations, an ED assessment would explore a wide variety of issues, including Elena's beliefs about body shape and weight, specific eating behaviors, reliance on purging behaviors, mood instability, safety concerns, past psychiatric treatment, family history of mental illness, and mental status changes. Collateral history from family members, partners, outside medical providers, or employers is often needed to obtain the most accurate picture, especially in patients like Elena who may minimize or deny their problems.

Clinicians who work with individuals with co-occurring EDs and SUDs may need to be unusually prepared to assess and manage medical issues. For example, apparent EDs can also be caused by mechanical gastrointestinal disorders or endocrine abnormalities (e.g., insulinoma, hyperthyroidism). Clinicians would generally measure and record an accurate height, weight, and BMI, which is beyond the typical activity of a therapist. Laboratory and diagnostic tests can assist in making the diagnosis and can help screen for dangerous metabolic complications that can result from purging and malnutrition. Patients with co-occurring ED and alcohol use disorder are more likely to present with significantly elevated levels of hepatic transaminases, especially when acutely malnourished. Female patients should always receive a pregnancy test, particularly when there are complaints of amenorrhea, frequent vomiting, or rapid weight fluctuation, even if there is a previously documented ED.

Ruling out these potential medical concerns at the onset of treatment will help reduce misdiagnosis and can help guide treatment. For example, if there is evidence of an acute electrolyte abnormality (i.e., low potassium with purging, low sodium with excessive water intake), arrhythmia on the electrocardiogram, end-organ failure, or symptomatic hypotension and bradycardia, an inpatient hospitalization may be required. In regard to Elena, her history of excessive vomiting, recurrent food restriction, and likely dehydration could prompt an inpatient hospitalization to stabilize her prior to an outpatient treatment. Of note, patients who would commonly present with hypotension or bradycardia when malnourished may initially show normal to mildly elevated vital sign readings when in acute substance withdrawal; in this case, a "masked" rise in blood pressure may mislead clinicians into undertreating the alcohol withdrawal.

## PSYCHOTHERAPEUTIC AND PSYCHOSOCIAL INTERVENTIONS

Treatment should initially be focused on medical complications to both the ED and the SUD. Assuming the patient is safe to be treated as an outpatient, a crucial initial part of the treatment is an assessment of the patient's motivation. For example, Elena might benefit from an intensive residential or day treatment program to address her co-occurring disorders; as it stands, however, she is barely willing to attend a weekly psychotherapy and has not yet described having a problem or an interest in changing her behavior. It can also be critical to explore the patient's family and social supports, since these can be vital to both the therapy and the stability of the home environment.

Cognitive-behavioral therapy (CBT) is the most typical psychotherapy used in addressing co-occurring EDs and SUDs (Dunn et al. 2006). CBT helps establish a pattern of self-monitoring so that the patient can identify precipitants for dysfunctional behavior and draw connections among thoughts, feelings and behaviors. Motivational interviewing may also be useful at the start of CBT to enhance patient commitment to sobriety, although use of a more systematized motivational approach, such as motivational enhancement therapy (MET), has shown mixed results with little change in treatment compliance over time (Dunn et al. 2006). There has also been emerging interest in the use of dialectical behavioral therapy (DBT) to target the emotional dysregulation and coping instability seen at the intersection of bulimia nervosa, binge-eating disorder, and substance abuse. Early studies comparing the effectiveness of DBT with a mix of CBT and motivational approaches ("treatment as usual" group) have been promising, suggesting that DBT leads to more consistent improvement in depressive symptoms, frequency of substance use, and rebound from negative emotions at both 3- and 6-month follow-ups (Courbasson et al. 2012). Use of DBT may be associated with improvements in binge-purge symptoms and sobriety even when these symptoms are not addressed directly in the therapy, highlighting the potential role of maladaptive coping patterns in perpetuating both disorders (Agras et al. 2000).

Many patients may find additional benefit from 12-step programs such as Alcoholics Anonymous. AA can run concurrently with the above psychotherapeutic interventions and provide daily, structured outpatient supports that can help maintain sobriety.

## PHARMACOLOGICAL CONSIDERATIONS

Psychotherapy is generally the core therapeutic intervention for co-occurring EDs and SUDs, but adjunctive psychotropic medication may maximize treatment outcomes. In many cases, the combination of pharmacological agents and evidence-based psychotherapies can be superior to the use of either treatment alone (Wilson 1996).

Selective serotonin reuptake inhibitors (SSRIs), such as fluoxetine, are often effective in limiting the intensity of purging behaviors in BN and alleviating the depression that may initiate or maintain patterns of disordered eating. Since depressive features, in particular, often complicate the course of both binge-purge and SUDs, SSRIs are often used at the onset of a treatment (Grilo et al. 2002). SSRIs may also be one of the safest medication options for this patient population given their low side-effect profile relative to other agents and lack of abuse potential.

Medications have proven consistently ineffective in the treatment of AN. Antidepressants, including fluoxetine, have been most studied, likely because of the depression, anxiety, and obsessionality symptoms associated with the disorder. Despite the symptomatic overlap between AN and other conditions that respond to antidepressant medications, fluoxetine is not associated with benefit compared with placebo in this clinical group (Attia et al. 1998).

There is emerging support for the use of second-generation antipsychotic medications such as olanzapine to target weight restoration and some associated psychological symptoms in AN (Lebow et al. 2013). The role for antipsychotic medications in combined treatment of ED and SUD is not yet fully understood, though second-generation antipsychotics are preferred to first-generation agents because of the former's more favorable side-effect profile as well as a potential reduction in substance cravings (American Psychiatric Association 2013). Second-generation antipsychotic medications are also used in detox and other outpatient settings to address symptoms of mood instability or insomnia, especially because other sedating medications, such as benzodiazepines, can be problematic in patients with SUDs.

Clinicians should also consider medication-assisted treatments for SUDs (e.g., naltrexone for alcohol use disorder and buprenorphine for opioid use disorder), although there will be special considerations for individuals with EDs. For example, bupropion is a first-line medication for smoking cessation and can be quite effective in curbing substance cravings. It can also function as a useful alternative to SSRIs or tricyclic antidepressants when combating the depressive and amotivational features tied to EDs and SUDs. Despite these positive attributes, bupropion's use in treating low-weight patients is relatively contraindicated because there is a significant risk of seizures (the combination of medication and malnutrition can significantly lower one's seizure threshold). Of note, patients with AN may request this medication despite its side effects because it is also known to be an effective appetite suppressant.

Table 9–1 lists other medications that may be encountered clinically at the nexus of ED and SUD treatments, each offering unique risks and benefits.

# Conclusion

Successful treatment of co-occurring EDs and SUDs requires the development of a tactful alliance and the use of multiple treatment strategies. The case of Elena is typical of a subset of these patients in that she appears to have developed an alcohol use disorder in the context of BN, though both seem to have developed in the context of the stresses of her first year of college. Although evidence is limited, it appears that the combination of psychotherapy (such as CBT or DBT) and medication may prove best for the combination of binge-purge symptoms and substance abuse, while AN and the restricting disorders are often initially treated by behavioral psychotherapies without medication and through the development of structured support.

## KEY POINTS

- Patients with eating disorders (EDs) may abuse a variety of substances to aid in weight loss, suppress appetite, or relieve feelings of fullness, ranging from nonprescription laxative medications to illicit drugs.

- Studies indicate that the presence of a preexisting ED will more likely be associated with the later development of substance use disorders (SUDs) than the other way around.

**TABLE 9–1.** Commonly encountered medications in treatments for eating disorders and substance use disorders

| Drug category | Common agents | Negatives | Positives |
|---|---|---|---|
| SSRIs | Fluoxetine Escitalopram | No significant benefit over placebo in treatment of AN. Side effects of weight gain and fatigue may deter patients. Often underdosed for BN/BED in primary care settings (higher doses often needed; e.g., fluoxetine 60–80 mg/day). | Strong evidence of benefit for BN, BED, and SUD with improved impulsivity and mood. Less overall side effect risk compared with other mood agents. |
| SNRIs and atypical antidepressants | Bupropion (SR/XR) Venlafaxine XR | Bupropion is contraindicated in AN with lowered seizure threshold; may be abused for appetite-suppression side effects in all eating disorders. SNRIs can exacerbate nausea and dry mouth, especially in underweight patients. | SNRIs are potentially helpful for depression in BN/BED and SUD if no response to SSRIs. Bupropion is FDA-approved for smoking cessation and can help curb substance cravings. |
| Benzodiazepines | Alprazolam Clonazepam Lorazepam Diazepam | Exacerbate dizziness, orthostatic hypotension, and cognitive impairment when individual is malnourished. Often misused for self-treating anxiety in lieu of ED behavior or illicits/causes dependence. High seizure risk when purging is combined with benzodiazepine withdrawal. | When taken as prescribed for emergency symptoms, can be an effective treatment for panic disorder and GAD (commonly comorbid with EDs and SUDs). |

**TABLE 9–1.** Commonly encountered medications in treatments for eating disorders and substance use disorders (*continued*)

| Drug category | Common agents | Negatives | Positives |
|---|---|---|---|
| Stimulants | Amphetamine/ dextroamphet- amine (Adderall) IR, XR Methylphenidate (Ritalin/Concerta) Lisdexamfetamine (Vyvanse) | Misused for appetite suppression and concentration/energy boost (counters cognitive slowing and fatigue when indi- vidual is malnourished). Increases risk of arrhythmia in AN. Short-acting formula- tions can be abused like street stimulants (e.g., cocaine/methamphetamine). | Vyvanse was recently FDA-approved for reducing binge episodes in BED. Long-acting agents can help manage debilitating ADHD symptoms in SUD patients with less risk of abuse or diversion. |
| Opioid antagonists | Naltrexone | Early evidence shows limited benefit compared with placebo in reducing impulsive eating or binge symptoms in ED. Side effects of nausea can be severe and exacerbate impulses to purge. | Effective at reducing frequency of alcohol abuse and risk of relapse. Can reduce cravings for opiates and alcohol. Naltrexone can be clinically useful for comorbid pain disorders. |
| Mood stabilizers | Topiramate Lamotrigine Lithium Carbamazepine | Minimal benefit compared with placebo in managing weight loss and ED-specific behaviors. Topiramate is often abused for appetite suppression; cognitive dulling side effects may be pronounced in low- weight patients. Lithium may hasten complications of AN, such as renal dysfunction and hair loss. | Lamotrigine can be a good alternative for mood instability with limited risk of weight gain. Blood serum level of these agents can be monitored to ensure therapeutic dosing. Uniquely indicated for comorbid seizure disorders. |

**TABLE 9–1.** Commonly encountered medications in treatments for eating disorders and substance use disorders (*continued*)

| Drug category | Common agents | Negatives | Positives |
|---|---|---|---|
| Second-generation antipsychotics | Olanzapine Risperidone Quetiapine Ziprasidone | Patients often avoid use with widely reported side effect of weight gain. May cause excessive sedation. Can cause undesired appetite stimulation in BN/BED patients. Ziprasidone may increase risk of prolonged QTc interval on ECG in cardiac-vulnerable AN patients. | Emerging studies (of olanzapine in particular) suggest positive treatment effects for AN and OCD-traits. Side effect of weight gain can be useful in early treatment. These agents may act as effective mood stabilizers for binge-eating/purging type of AD in the context of ED and SUD. |

*Note.*    AN=anorexia nervosa; BED=binge-eating disorder; BN=bulimia nervosa; ECG=electrocardiogram; ED=eating disorder; FDA = U.S. Food and Drug Administration; GAD = generalized anxiety disorder; IR=immediate release; OCD=obsessive-compulsive disorder; SNRI=serotonin-norepinephrine reuptake inhibitor; SR = sustained release; SSRI=selective serotonin reuptake inhibitor; SUD=substance use disorder; XR=sustained release/extended release.

- The confluence of factors that lead to the development of an ED represents a "perfect storm" of environmental, genetic, and neurobiological factors that are qualitatively different from the dopamine-driven, neural pathway toward "rewards" that is seen in addiction-focused disorders.

- There is consistent support for the efficacy of CBT in early treatment, both self-directed and alongside therapist, in addressing behaviors that overlap between these two conditions. Evidence is also accumulating for the use of DBT strategies to improve impulsive coping patterns, and in particular with the binge-eating/purging type.

- Selective serotonin reuptake inhibitors are a treatment of choice in combination with psychotherapy for bulimia nervosa in the context of comorbid SUDs. In contrast, antidepressants have been seen to offer little to no benefit compared with placebo in anorexia nervosa.

# Questions

1. Which of the following contributes to the high prevalence of tobacco abuse in eating disorders (EDs)?

   A. Tobacco is notorious for suppressing appetite.
   B. Advertising for cigarettes has historically been associated with excessive eating.
   C. Smoking is more commonly seen in the restricting type of EDs.
   D. Tobacco use is associated with eating solid foods in social settings.

2. Which medication is commonly used in the management of substance use disorders (SUDs) but may be contraindicated in anorexia nervosa (AN)?

   A. Topiramate.
   B. Bupropion.
   C. Naltrexone.
   D. Citalopram.

3. Which one of the following evidence-based psychotherapy approaches would be most ideal when first approaching a 31-year-old

patient who is of low to average weight, purging multiple days per week, and struggling with intermittent heroin abuse?

A. Psychodynamic psychotherapy, followed by antidepressant trial.
B. Motivational interviewing, followed by a trial of cognitive-behavioral therapy (CBT) or dialectical behavioral therapy (DBT).
C. Family-based treatment (FBT) alone.
D. 12-step group program for BN.

# References

Agras WS, Walsh T, Fairburn CG, et al: A multicenter comparison of cognitive-behavioral therapy and interpersonal psychotherapy for bulimia nervosa. Arch Gen Psychiatry 57(5):459–466, 2000 10807486

American Psychiatric Association: Diagnostic and Statistical Manual of Mental Disorders, 5th Edition. Arlington, VA, American Psychiatric Association, 2013

Attia E, Haiman C, Walsh BT, et al: Does fluoxetine augment the inpatient treatment of anorexia nervosa? Am J Psychiatry 155(4):548–551, 1998 9546003

Barbarich-Marsteller NC, Foltin RW, Walsh BT: Does anorexia nervosa resemble an addiction? Curr Drug Abuse Rev 4(3):197–200, 2011 21999694

Courbasson C, Nishikawa Y, Dixon L: Outcome of dialectical behaviour therapy for concurrent eating and substance use disorders. Clin Psychol Psychother 19(5):434–449, 2012 21416557

Dunn EC, Neighbors C, Larimer ME: Motivational enhancement therapy and self-help treatment for binge eaters. Psychol Addict Behav 20(1):44–52, 2006 16536664

Franko DL, Dorer DJ, Keel PK, et al: How do eating disorders and alcohol use disorder influence each other? Int J Eat Disord 38(3):200–207, 2005 16216020

Gregorowski C, Seedat S, Jordaan GP: A clinical approach to the assessment and management of co-morbid eating disorders and substance use disorders. BMC Psychiatry 13:289, 2013 24200300

Grilo CM, Sinha R, O'Malley SS: Eating disorders and alcohol use disorders. National Institute on Alcohol Abuse and Alcoholism, November 2002. Available at: https://pubs.niaaa.nih.gov/publications/arh26-2/151-160.htm. Accessed February 7, 2017.

Jeffers A, Benotsch EG, Koester S: Misuse of prescription stimulants for weight loss, psychosocial variables, and eating disordered behaviors. Appetite 65:8–13, 2013 23376413

Krug I, Treasure J, Anderluh M, et al: Present and lifetime comorbidity of tobacco, alcohol and drug use in eating disorders: a European multicenter study. Drug Alcohol Depend 97(1-2):169–179, 2008 18571341

Lebow J, Sim LA, Erwin PJ, Murad MH: The effect of atypical antipsychotic medications in individuals with anorexia nervosa: a systematic review and meta-analysis. Int J Eat Disord 46(4):332–339, 2013 23001863

Mitchell JE, Specker S, Edmonson K: Management of substance abuse and dependence, in Handbook of Treatment for Eating Disorders, 2nd Edition. Edited by Garner DM, Garfield PE. New York, Guilford, 1997, pp 415–423

National Center on Addiction and Substance Abuse at Columbia University: Food for thought: substance abuse and eating disorders. 2003. Available at: http://www.centeronaddiction.org/addiction-research/reports/food-thought-substance-abuse-and-eating-disorders. Accessed February 6, 2017.

Powers PS: Management of patients with comorbid medical conditions, in Handbook of Treatment for Eating Disorders, 2nd Edition. Edited by Garner DM, Garfield PE. New York, Guilford, 1997, pp 424–436

Root TL, Pisetsky EM, Thornton L, et al: Patterns of co-morbidity of eating disorders and substance use in Swedish females. Psychol Med 40(1):105–115, 2010 19379530

Stock SL, Goldberg E, Corbett S, Katzman DK: Substance use in female adolescents with eating disorders. J Adolesc Health 31(2):176–182, 2002 12127388

Wilson GT: Treatment of bulimia nervosa: when CBT fails. Behav Res Ther 34(3):197–212, 1996 8881090

# 10

# GAMBLING DISORDER

*Mayumi Okuda, M.D.*
*Silvia Franco, M.D.*
*Ariel Kor, Ph.D.*

The inclusion of gambling disorder (GD) within the DSM-5 chapter that otherwise focuses on substance use disorders (SUDs) reflects their many shared qualities, including the distress and dysfunction arising from problematic behavior. In addition, there is much overlap between the two disorders, so that roughly half of people with GD will also have a SUD, most often alcohol use disorder (Blanco et al. 2015; Petry et al. 2005). Individuals with *both* GD and SUD are at greater risk of interpersonal difficulties, legal problems, financial losses, physical health problems, and suicidality (Cowlishaw and Hakes 2015; Kim et al. 2016).

In this chapter, we present a case of a man with GD and alcohol use disorder. We discuss typical diagnostic difficulties, including how best to approach patients who are often not transparently forthcoming about their symptoms. We then describe treatment issues that include family involvement, cognitive-behavioral strategies, the importance of developing an integrated strategy rather than treating only one diagnosis, and typical barriers to effectiveness. While these clinical points are applied to the particular case, the general principles can be applied to patients with GD and a variety of other SUDs.

## Clinical Case

Peter is a 39-year-old man who is married and has three children. At the time of the initial intake, Peter had been working as a vice president at a leading consulting firm. He presented for treatment at a clinic after having been given an ultimatum by his wife, who was threatening to get a divorce. She had been dissatisfied with their marriage for several years. Concerned that he was having an affair, she searched his computer and discovered a hidden file that neatly laid out his long-standing gambling losses. She also discovered that he had spent their entire savings and emptied their retirement account. In addition, they now owed a total of $80,000 to five "secret" credit cards. At that point, his wife had told him to get help or move out.

At the time of the evaluation, Peter denied other psychiatric complaints, medical illnesses, and substance abuse. He described himself as a "social drinker" but added that both his parents were "probably alcoholics" who had often been abusive to him and to each other when drunk. On exam, Peter was dressed impeccably and was calm, coherent, and without any confusion, suicidality, or cognitive decline.

Peter said he began gambling by buying scratch cards as a child. In college, he played poker regularly and occasionally made small sports bets. During and after business school, he continued the sports betting, adding that the bets helped him deal with the stress of school and then with his work as a business consultant and his marriage to a woman he had met in business school. His gambling escalated following the death of his mother and the births of his three children. Even though his house was "full of people," the screaming kids made him increasingly retreat to his basement office (which he called his "man cave"), where he studied sports and also felt increasingly isolated and anxious. While he had initially bet small amounts of money on a few games per month, he began to bet larger amounts, often during the day. While he was "obsessed" with sports statistics and often watched sports commentary during a typical workday, he was very successful at work through his early 30s.

In recent years, Peter's gambling appears to have become more problematic, leading to a variety of compensatory activities. After big losses, Peter would focus on finding a high-risk bet that would win back his money. Whether at work or at home, he found himself increasingly anxious and irritable, especially when interrupted while watching television and doing his online sports research. He found his wife and children to be especially annoying, especially since none of them appeared to understand the stress he was under. On several occasions, he had tried to stop betting on games by disabling smartphone applications and blocking sports Web sites, but he had generally regained access within a few hours.

When his wife confronted him with the computer information, Peter initially tried to argue with her. Within a day, however, he had made the appointment with a psychiatrist.

GD was the most clear diagnosis for Peter. He also had prominent anxiety that seemed to have a complicated relationship with the gambling. Although Peter said he had initially gambled to reduce anxiety, much of his current anxiety appeared to be related to the mounting financial losses and ongoing stress regarding his family and work. It was not clear whether the anxiety warranted a specific therapeutic focus. Peter also described "social drinking" and had a strong family history of alcohol use disorder, but he insisted alcohol was not a problem. Peter displayed criminal financial behavior, and his empathy for his wife and children appeared limited, but, as with the substance use disorders, DSM-5 counsels to avoid a diagnosis of antisocial personality disorder when the antisocial behaviors involve the addiction.

One of the first tasks of treatment was to conduct a "functional analysis" of the gambling, in which the individual is asked to describe his gambling activities in detail. Peter identified his gambling triggers, which included anxiety and the great pleasure he felt when he won (or at least the pleasure he had initially felt when he won; he realized that in recent months or years, he tended to respond to winning bets with a grim thought that he should have bet more money on the winners). Peter described his pride in knowing so much about sports; this knowledge had initially led him to feeling a sense of camaraderie with other men, though he acknowledged that while he had originally spent a lot of time in sports bars, he had recently spent long hours alone in the basement, researching online data, listening to a cable sports network, and rarely watching a game in its entirety. He described his ongoing confusion and anger that he could be such a "loser" when he was so well prepared, and added that while he knew that he needed help, he was still confident that he could "crack the system" and win back his money.

This initial phase had several goals, including the development of an alliance so that Peter could feel understood and be willing to continue the treatment. In addition, an initial focus was to identify irrational beliefs. In Peter's case, a core irrational belief was his conviction that sports betting is a game of skill that can be mastered through intelligence, effort, and an understanding of statistics. Such irrational beliefs can play a powerful role in maintaining the dysfunctional behavior and in triggering relapses during the treatment.

After much debate, Peter agreed to let his wife gain sole control over their finances. He cancelled his credit cards and changed his phone number so that he could not be contacted by bookies. He refrained from watching sports and even consented to locking the door to his basement office. After a few weeks of abstinence, Peter experienced a relapse, where he gambled after going to a sports bar when he traveled to visit some friends.

As the alliance deepened, Peter acknowledged that he abused alcohol. He had a "few drinks" daily and drank until blacking out when traveling or particularly stressed. While intoxicated, he tended to place unusually large bets and also engaged in recurrent, compulsive sexual activities. Facilitated by a smartphone app, Peter reported spending several hours a day flirting with strangers and averaging two or three sexual encounters with different women each week. As with the gambling and alcohol, he felt ashamed but was unable to control his sexual behavior.

The development of a more thorough history allowed the therapy to focus on multiple issues. His alcohol use disorder became an additional focus of treatment. Motivational interviewing, naltrexone, and referral to Alcoholics Anonymous led to prolonged abstinence from alcohol, which appeared to reduce the number and intensity of his gambling relapses. In addition, Peter avoided other triggers. The family cancelled their subscription to cable television so that Peter couldn't easily watch all-day sports. His wife continued to manage their money. To deal with his tendency to obsess over the specifics, he wasn't allowed even to have access to the online bank statements without his wife present. Peter chose a job that required no traveling, which reduced his unsupervised time. He also stopped taking solo vacations during times when there would be major sporting events on weekday television (e.g., March Madness and the Olympics). Instead, he and his wife scheduled time for them to be together and for him to spend time with their children. His current treatment is focused on relapse prevention and paying off his debt.

# Discussion

It is clear that Peter has a diagnosis of GD. As part of a comprehensive psychiatric evaluation for an individual with any behavioral addiction, it is crucial to rule out conditions such as mood, anxiety, and personality disorders, or other SUDs, that can either explain or worsen the patient's condition. It is also important to consider other types of gambling in the differential diagnosis (Table 10–1). As evidenced in the case, Peter also has comorbid alcohol use disorder that contributes to his presentation. It is worth mentioning that if an individual's symptoms meet criteria for both GD and a SUD, clinicians should diagnose both rather than attribute one to the other; even if one disorder is predominant, each disorder should be addressed in treatment.

GD is diagnosed following DSM-5 criteria (American Psychiatric Association 2013) (Box 10–1). Some of the major changes in this disorder from DSM-IV to DSM-5 include 1) renaming "Pathological Gambling" as "Gambling Disorder"; 2) eliminating the criterion "committing illegal acts such as forgery, fraud, theft, or embezzlement to finance gambling"; 3) lowering the threshold for diagnosis from 5 out of 10 criteria to 4 out of 9 criteria; and 4) including gambling disorder among the SUDs. Data reported in this chapter are based on studies using the DSM-IV classification of pathological gambling and problem gambling (subthreshold pathological gambling), and the term gambling disorder, or GD, is used to denote both pathological and problem gambling. As described in the case, Peter's presentation meets all the criteria for GD, including preoccupation and persistent thoughts about his gambling; restlessness and irritability when attempting to cut down on his gambling; unsuccessful attempts to control his gambling; gambling with increasing amounts of money; gambling when feeling distressed; after losing, returning the next day to get even (chasing losses); lying to his family and friends about the extent of his gambling; jeopardizing relationships and job opportunities; and relying on others to relieve desperate financial situations caused by gambling. These and other phenomenological characteristics share similarities with those of SUDs: craving or urges, loss of control (chasing losses), withdrawal symptoms (restlessness or irritability), tolerance (betting increasing amounts of money), repeated unsuccessful attempts to stop the behavior, and a compulsive pursuit of the behavior despite its serious negative consequences.

---

**TABLE 10–1.  Differential diagnosis for gambling disorder (GD)**

| | |
|---|---|
| Social gambling | Individuals who gamble socially/recreationally are able to limit and control their gambling activities without exhibiting symptoms of GD. |
| Gambling associated with bipolar disorder | Excessive gambling exclusively occurring in the context of a manic episode is not considered GD, as this is better explained by a diagnosis of bipolar disorder. Symptoms of GD in these patients should diminish when symptoms of mania or hypomania subside. Nonetheless, GD can still be diagnosed in patients with bipolar disorder if symptoms persist outside of the context of a manic episode (e.g., during a depressive episode). |
| Professional gambling | Some individuals support themselves financially by engaging in gambling activities that require skill and chance (e.g., poker) without developing GD. However, those who display progressive and maladaptive gambling behaviors may be diagnosed with a GD. |
| GD related to use of dopaminergic agents | Compulsive gambling and other behavioral addictions are a serious and increasingly recognized complication of dopamine replacement therapy in Parkinson's disease and restless legs syndrome. The most commonly implicated agents are pramipexole and ropinirole. GD symptoms appear to improve or often resolve after reducing or discontinuing the dopamine agent when this is possible (Weintraub and Nirenberg 2013). |

---

Box 10–1.    DSM-5 Diagnostic Criteria for Gambling Disorder

A. Persistent and recurrent problematic gambling behavior leading to clinically significant impairment or distress, as indicated by the individual exhibiting four (or more) of the following in a 12-month period:

1. Needs to gamble with increasing amounts of money in order to achieve the desired excitement.
2. Is restless or irritable when attempting to cut down or stop gambling.
3. Has made repeated unsuccessful efforts to control, cut back, or stop gambling.

4. Is often preoccupied with gambling (e.g., having persistent thoughts of reliving past gambling experiences, handicapping or planning the next venture, thinking of ways to get money with which to gamble).
5. Often gambles when feeling distressed (e.g., helpless, guilty, anxious, depressed).
6. After losing money gambling, often returns another day to get even ("chasing" one's losses).
7. Lies to conceal the extent of involvement with gambling.
8. Has jeopardized or lost a significant relationship, job, or educational or career opportunity because of gambling.
9. Relies on others to provide money to relieve desperate financial situations caused by gambling.

B. The gambling behavior is not better explained by a manic episode.

*Specify* if:

**Episodic:** Meeting diagnostic criteria at more than one time point, with symptoms subsiding between periods of gambling disorder for at least several months.

**Persistent:** Experiencing continuous symptoms, to meet diagnostic criteria for multiple years.

*Specify* if:

**In early remission:** After full criteria for gambling disorder were previously met, none of the criteria for gambling disorder have been met for at least 3 months but for less than 12 months.

**In sustained remission:** After full criteria for gambling disorder were previously met, none of the criteria for gambling disorder have been met during a period of 12 months or longer.

*Specify* current severity:

**Mild:** 4–5 criteria met.

**Moderate:** 6–7 criteria met.

**Severe:** 8–9 criteria met.

A large epidemiological survey conducted in the United States (Petry et al. 2005) found that the prevalence of GD was 1% among individuals with alcohol use disorder and 1.6% among those with any SUD. On the other hand, among individuals with GD, 73% had an alcohol use disorder, 38% had a non-alcohol SUD, and 60% had nicotine dependence. In treatment-seeking populations, around 4.3% of individuals with SUD have a lifetime GD and an additional 7.2% endorse criteria along the spectrum of GD (three to five DSM-IV symptoms) (Cowlishaw and Hakes 2015). In at least one methadone maintenance program, 21% of patients had symptoms that met the criteria for GD, with 65% of them having the onset of GD within 2 years of the onset of their SUD (Spunt et al. 1998).

Risk factors associated with the development of GD include male gender, initiation of gambling at an early age, childhood adverse events, being a member of a racial/ethnic minority group, living in close proximity to a gambling venue, low socioeconomic status, impulsivity, psychiatric comorbidity, and a family history of GD or SUDs (Blanco et al. 2015). As exemplified in this case, Peter's early onset of gambling behavior may have predisposed him to GD in adulthood, mirroring consequences of early onset of substance use. As with SUD, GD tends to have a chronic course with either continuous episodic patterns or periods of abstinence of variable duration (weeks to years) followed by lapses (e.g., gambling 1 day after a period of abstinence) or full blown relapses (e.g., return to a cycle of gambling habits after a period of abstinence). Most individuals have a gradual development of their gambling problems, with the problematic gambling taking several years to progress to a diagnosis of GD. In some cases, GD can develop shortly after gambling initiation—a pattern that is more commonly seen in machine gamblers (Breen and Zimmerman 2002). First described in alcohol use disorder, the course of GD in women has also been described as starting gambling later in life but having a shorter period between recreational and problematic gambling ("telescoping phenomenon").

GD and SUDs may affect each other through different pathways. SUD may play a role in the initiation, maintenance, or worsening of an existing GD. Several studies demonstrate that individuals are more likely to gamble when under the influence of moderate doses of alcohol than when taking placebo (Kyngdon and Dickerson 1999). Many gambling activities are accompanied by alcohol use (e.g., casinos providing free alcohol to patrons, betting in sports bars), making simultaneous gambling and alcohol consumption a frequent activity (Petry et al. 2005). Additionally, alcohol consumption paired with gambling is associated with larger average bets and more rapid money losses (Cronce and Corbin 2010).

Negative consequences appear to be more frequent among individuals that face both GD and SUD. For example, individuals with GD who drink in excess are at a significant higher risk for suicidal ideation (Kim et al. 2016). Cocaine use is also associated with higher levels of impulsive behavior, which is strongly correlated with GD and has been shown to impair decision making during a gambling task (Hulka et al. 2015). Likewise, the prevalence of other psychiatric disorders, such as mood, anxiety, or personality disorders, has been shown to be significantly higher in individuals with both GD and alcohol use disorder than in individuals with GD only. GD may be one of many risky behaviors that individuals engage in during substance use. In the case presented, Peter also engages in risky sexual behaviors, including unprotected sex with strangers. It is well known that drug consumption can facilitate such high-risk behaviors (Stall and Leigh 1994).

The association between GD and SUD suggests there may be common etiological factors that contribute to both of these disorders (Blanco et al. 2015; Frascella et al. 2010). Disturbances in several neurotransmitter systems, including the noradrenaline (arousal and excitement), serotonin (behavior initiation and cessation), dopamine (reward and reinforcement), and opioid (pleasure and urges) systems, appear to influence both behavioral addictions and SUDs. Other commonalities include findings in brain imaging data (e.g., alterations in reward circuit; poor frontal regulation during exposure to a gambling scenario/substance abuse cues) and high heritability (Frascella et al. 2010). Familial and twin studies have reported a higher prevalence of GD in family members of individuals diagnosed with GD, suggesting that familial transmission may play a role in the etiology of GD. Studies conducted in clinical samples have reported a lifetime prevalence of GD of up to 20% among first-degree relatives of individuals with GD (Walters 2001). Two twin studies have also provided evidence of the role of genetic factors in the development of GD (Slutske et al. 2000). Genetic influences appear to account for 49% of the variation in liability for GD, and there has not been evidence of gender differences in this variation. Importantly, it also appears that GD and alcohol use disorder have common genetic underpinnings. These two twin studies also demonstrated that overlapping genetic risk factors account for more than half of the association in the risk for GD and alcohol use disorder in both men and women (Slutske et al. 2000). As exemplified in this case, while Peter did not have any other family members with GD, both of his parents had a history of alcohol use disorder.

Peter also appears to have "compulsive sexual behavior," which is also known as "hypersexuality" or "sexual addiction." People with compulsive sexual behavior, though this is not an approved diagnosis within DSM-5, appear to make up a recognizable group of persons with similar features: inappropriate or excessive sexual fantasies, urges, cravings or behaviors that generate subjective distress or impairment in daily functioning (Kor et al. 2013). These fantasies, urges, cravings, or behaviors may increase over time and have been linked to impairments in health and psychosocial and interpersonal functioning (Kor et al. 2013). Given its damaging effects on his life, Peter's sexual behavior warrants clinical attention, though it is also likely reduction of gambling triggers such as alcohol and travel may be enough to reduce the compulsive sexual behavior as well.

There are many barriers to appropriate treatment for patients with co-occurring GD and SUDs. GD is often unrecognized and not typically assessed. There are several available instruments to screen for GD, including the Structured Clinical Interview for Pathological Gambling (SCI-PG; Grant et al. 2004), the South Oaks Gambling Screen (SOGS; Lesieur and Blume 1987), the Diagnostic Interview for Gambling Severity (DIGS; Winters et al. 2002), the Gamblers Anonymous 20 Questions (Derevensky and Gupta 2000), the Massachusetts Gambling Screen (MAGS; Shaffer et al. 1994), and the Gambling Assessment Module (GAM-IV; Cunningham-Williams et al. 2000, 2003), among many others. The Lie/Bet Questionnaire (Johnson et al. 1997) is a simple and brief screening tool that includes two questions that are identified as the best predictors for GD: "Have you ever had to lie to people important to you about how much you gambled?" "Have you ever felt the need to bet more and more money?"

Continued research of the neurobiological alterations in individuals with behavioral disorders, and its correlation with SUDs, will likely improve our understanding and implementation of better prevention and treatment strategies to help this population.

# Treatment

## PSYCHOTHERAPEUTIC AND PSYCHOSOCIAL INTERVENTIONS

During the initial phase of treatment, it would be useful to clarify that Peter may or may not view alcohol as an independent problem but that it is clearly implicated in his gambling. Given that interaction, both should be the subject of clinical attention (Table 10–2).

Cognitive-behavioral therapy (CBT) has been proven to be the most efficacious treatment for GD. In this case presentation, Peter presented to care seeking treatment for his GD, and he did not identify alcohol as a major issue. CBT for GD focuses on achieving abstinence from gambling through the acquisition of skills that facilitate lifestyle changes and restructure the environment to increase reinforcement from nongambling behaviors. As depicted in this case, and as part of the components of CBT treatment, Peter's therapist encouraged him to describe his gambling activities, helping him to identify triggers for gambling and focus on the places, times, activities, moods, and people with whom he was

**TABLE 10–2.** Treatment tips

Cognitive-behavioral therapy is the most effective treatment for gambling disorder (GD) and may address co-occurring disorders as well.

Pharmacological interventions should be directed toward treating the co-occurring disorder(s) given the lack of evidence for medications for GD.

Opioid antagonists (naltrexone and nalmefene) have shown some promise in small randomized trials.

more likely to gamble. In this scenario, the therapist noted that while Peter felt very motivated to abstain from gambling, he was ambivalent about his alcohol use. Motivational interviewing (MI) has been shown to be useful in treating SUDs. MI, as either a stand-alone treatment or in the form of motivational enhancement combined with CBT, has also been shown to decrease gambling frequency and increase the likelihood of remission from GD. Therefore, in view of the patient's ambivalence toward his alcohol use, the therapist wisely employed MI to help move the patient toward change and accept treatment for his alcohol use disorder.

## PHARMACOLOGICAL INTERVENTIONS

An additional component of treatment in this case was the use of a pharmacological agent. To date, there are no medications approved by the U.S. Food and Drug Administration (FDA) for GD. While several medications, including selective serotonin reuptake inhibitors, bupropion, lithium, olanzapine and topiramate have been tested in open-label or small, randomized controlled trials, some of these trials have yielded mixed results or have been limited by small samples or short follow-up. Opioid antagonists (naltrexone and nalmefene) have shown effectiveness in small randomized trials. Replication in larger, randomized controlled trials with long-term follow-up is needed before definitive recommendations can be made. Therefore, choice of medication may be most effective when directed toward the patient's comorbid psychiatric disorder, which could include SUDs, mood or anxiety disorders, and attention-deficit/ hyperactivity disorder, which frequently co-occur in patients with GD. In this particular case, the patient's symptoms met the criteria for an alcohol use disorder for which the opioid receptor antagonist naltrexone is indicated. Naltrexone has been found to reduce alcohol consumption compared with placebo in several randomized clinical trials for alcohol dependence. Secondary analyses of two double-blind placebo-controlled trials testing naltrexone and nalmefene found that a positive family history of alcohol use disorders was the strongest predictor of response to opiate antagonists (Grant et al. 2008b). Furthermore, an open-label and two small randomized, placebo-controlled trials (Grant et al. 2008a) suggest that naltrexone may result in reduction of gambling symptoms. These findings should be interpreted with caution, given the high placebo-response rates and high dropout rates found in GD studies examining naltrexone. However, given the indication of naltrexone for alcohol use disorder in this patient and the preliminary findings of possible effects on GD, naltrexone might be specifically helpful in reducing persistent gambling urges. Contrary to a common clinical perception, individuals whose SUD is in remisison have a lower likelihood of developing another SUD (Blanco et al. 2014). Thus, treating this patient's GD and alcohol use disorder simultaneously likely contributed to improved clinical outcomes.

# Conclusion

SUDs, particularly alcohol use disorder, are common among individuals with GD. Peter's case illustrates how both disorders can contribute to the perpetuation of each other and the rationale for treating them simultaneously. Fortunately, there are several commonalities in terms of treatments for these two conditions, including evidence supporting the use of psychotherapeutic interventions like CBT and MI, and some promising pharmacological treatments that could address both addictions. Knowledge on the prevalence and treatment of other proposed behavioral addictions, such as compulsive sexual disorder, is lacking.

## KEY POINTS

- DSM-5 now includes gambling disorder in the chapter "Substance-Related and Addictive Disorders."
- The new definition of GD has eliminated the criterion "committing illegal acts such as forgery, fraud, theft, or embezzlement to finance gambling."
- More than half of all patients with GD have a concurrent substance use disorder (SUD), with alcohol use disorder being the most prevalent.
- Patients with co-occurring GD and SUDs have worse clinical outcomes compared with those with GD but without a SUD.

- Use of cognitive-behavioral therapy (CBT) in the treatment of GD has the strongest evidence for efficacy.
- Use of psychopharmacological treatment for GD is being explored but requires further study.
- There are many similarities in treatment for GD and SUDs, with both conditions benefitting from CBT, motivational interviewing, and other pharmacological treatments, including opioid antagonists.

## Questions

1. Approximately what percentage of individuals with gambling disorder (GD) has any lifetime comorbid substance use disorder (SUD)?

    A. 5%–10%.
    B. 20%–30%.
    C. 40%–60%.
    D. More than 60%.

2. Which of the following is *true* regarding the comorbidity between GD and SUD?

    A. Patients with co-occurring GD and SUD have better clinical outcomes compared with those without a SUD.
    B. Alcohol consumption paired with gambling is associated with smaller average bets and less money lost.
    C. Withdrawal symptoms and tolerance are characteristic of SUDs and GD.
    D. The prevalence of other psychiatric disorders, such as mood, anxiety, or personality disorders, is significantly lower in individuals with both GD and SUD than in individuals with only GD.

3. Which of the following psychotherapeutic treatments is the most efficacious in the treatment of GD?

    A. Assertive community treatment (ACT).
    B. Cognitive-behavioral therapy (CBT).
    C. Contingency management.
    D. Dialectical behavioral therapy (DBT).

# References

American Psychiatric Association: Diagnostic and Statistical Manual of Mental Disorders, 5th Edition. Arlington, VA, American Psychiatric Association, 2013

Blanco C, Okuda M, Wang S, et al: Testing the drug substitution switching-addictions hypothesis: a prospective study in a nationally representative sample. JAMA Psychiatry 71(11):1246–1253, 2014 25208305

Blanco C, Hanania J, Petry NM, et al: Towards a comprehensive developmental model of pathological gambling. Addiction 110(8):1340–1351, 2015 25879250

Breen RB, Zimmerman M: Rapid onset of pathological gambling in machine gamblers. J Gambl Stud 18(1):31–43, 2002 12050846

Cowlishaw S, Hakes JK: Pathological and problem gambling in substance use treatment: results from the National Epidemiologic Survey on Alcohol and Related Conditions (NESARC). Am J Addict 24(5):467–474, 2015 25950376

Cronce JM, Corbin WR: Effects of alcohol and initial gambling outcomes on within-session gambling behavior. Exp Clin Psychopharmacol 18(2):145–157, 2010 20384426

Cunningham-Williams RM, Cottler LB, Mangiaforte S: The development of the Gambling Assessment Module (GAM-IV). Presented at the 11th International Conference on Gambling and Risk-Taking, Las Vegas, NV, June 12–16, 2000

Cunningham-Williams RM, Cottler LB, Books SJ: Gambling Assessment Module—Self-Administered (GAM-IV-S). St Louis, MO, Washington University School of Medicine, July 2001, revised July 2003

Derevensky JL, Gupta R: Prevalence estimates of adolescent gambling: a comparison of the SOGS-RA, DSM-IV-J, and the GA 20 questions. J Gambl Stud 16(2–3):227–251, 2000 14634314

Frascella J, Potenza MN, Brown LL, et al: Shared brain vulnerabilities open the way for nonsubstance addictions: carving addiction at a new joint? Ann N Y Acad Sci 1187:294–315, 2010 20201859

Grant JE, Steinberg MA, Kim SW, et al: Preliminary validity and reliability testing of a structured clinical interview for pathological gambling. Psychiatry Res 128(1):79–88, 2004 15450917

Grant JE, Kim SW, Hartman BK: A double-blind, placebo-controlled study of the opiate antagonist naltrexone in the treatment of pathological gambling urges. J Clin Psychiatry 69(5):783–789, 2008a 18384246

Grant JE, Kim SW, Hollander E, Potenza MN: Predicting response to opiate antagonists and placebo in the treatment of pathological gambling. Psychopharmacology (Berl) 200(4):521–527, 2008b 18581096

Hulka LM, Vonmoos M, Preller KH, et al: Changes in cocaine consumption are associated with fluctuations in self-reported impulsivity and gambling decision-making. Psychol Med 45(14):3097–3110, 2015 26081043

Johnson EE, Hamer R, Nora RM, et al: The Lie/Bet Questionnaire for screening pathological gamblers. Psychol Rep 80(1):83–88, 1997 9122356

Kim HS, Salmon M, Wohl MJ, et al: A dangerous cocktail: alcohol consumption increases suicidal ideations among problem gamblers in the general population. Addict Behav 55:50–55, 2016 26790140

Kor A, Fogel Y, Reid RC, et al: Should hypersexual disorder be classified as an addiction? Sex Addict Compulsivity 20(1–2):27–47, 2013 24273404

Kyngdon A, Dickerson M: An experimental study of the effect of prior alcohol consumption on a simulated gambling activity. Addiction 94(5):697–707, 1999 10563034

Lesieur HR, Blume SB: The South Oaks Gambling Screen (SOGS): a new instrument for the identification of pathological gamblers. Am J Psychiatry 144(9):1184–1188, 1987 3631315

Petry NM, Stinson FS, Grant BF: Comorbidity of DSM-IV pathological gambling and other psychiatric disorders: results from the National Epidemiologic Survey on Alcohol and Related Conditions. J Clin Psychiatry 66(5):564–574, 2005 15889941

Shaffer HJ, LaBrie R, Scanlan KM, Cummings TN: Pathological gambling among adolescents: Massachusetts Gambling Screen (MAGS). J Gambl Stud 10(4):339–362, 1994

Slutske WS, Eisen S, True WR, et al: Common genetic vulnerability for pathological gambling and alcohol dependence in men. Arch Gen Psychiatry 57(7):666–673, 2000 10891037

Spunt B, Dupont I, Lesieur H, et al: Pathological gambling and substance misuse: a review of the literature. Subst Use Misuse 33(13):2535–2560, 1998 9818989

Stall R, Leigh B: Understanding the relationship between drug or alcohol use and high risk sexual activity for HIV transmission: where do we go from here? Addiction 89(2):131–134, 1994 8173473

Walters GD: Behavior genetic research on gambling and problem gambling: a preliminary meta-analysis of available data. J Gambl Stud 17(4):255–271, 2001 11842524

Weintraub D, Nirenberg MJ: Impulse control and related disorders in Parkinson's disease. Neurodegener Dis 11:63–71, 2013 23038208

Winters KC, Specker S, Stinchfield R: Measuring pathological gambling with the Diagnostic Interview for Gambling Severity (DIGS), in The Downside: Problem and Pathological Gambling. Edited by Marotta JJ, Cornelius JA, Eadington WR. Reno, University of Nevada, 2002, pp 143–148

# PART 3

## SPECIFIC TREATMENTS

# 11

# TWELVE-STEP PROGRAMS

*Luke J. Archibald, M.D.*

Alcoholics Anonymous (AA), Narcotics Anonymous (NA), and other 12-step programs are widely available and effective treatments for individuals with and without co-occurring psychiatric disorders (CODs). While the literature supports the role of 12-step approaches for individuals with CODs, it appears that 12-step programs may be underutilized in this population. One reason for the underutilization is that some people with CODs may not be able to tolerate some aspects of 12-step programs; often, however, they can function fine when their more acute psychiatric symptoms are under control. A second reason is that some general-practice mental health practitioners may not be fully confident recommending a program with which they may not be completely familiar. Given the frequency of substance use disorders (SUDs) among people who present for mental health treatment, it behooves psychiatric clinicians to understand details of the 12-step programs so that they can confidently recommend and adapt the program to fit the needs of their patients.

Alcoholics Anonymous is a mutual-aid fellowship started in 1935 by Bill Wilson and Dr. Bob Smith. For at least 100 years prior to the founding of AA, other grassroots efforts to address alcoholism emerged but ultimately failed. AA now counts over 2 million members with more than 115,000 registered groups (Alcoholics Anonymous 1956; Nace 2014). Its primary purpose is "to carry its message to the alcoholic who still suffers." With other early members, Bill W. and Dr. Bob developed AA's 12-step program of spiritual and character development along with the 12 traditions to help the fellowship be stable and unified from outside influences (Alcoholics Anonymous 1978). Much of their work is available within literature published by AA, including the Big Book, which clarifies much of what is important to the AA program.

To "work the program" means to follow the 12 steps, attend meetings, work with a sponsor, and participate in the program. While one should review all the steps to familiarize oneself with AA concepts like "making amends" and "taking a personal inventory," consider the first two steps, which are often emphasized and debated. The first step involves admitting that one cannot control one's alcoholism, addiction, or compulsion. While this step may seem fairly obvious to the mental health clinician, many people spend a long time working on this particular step. Also, individuals with SUDs at times do not agree with the AA emphasis on powerlessness and complete abstinence, and prefer other programs like Moderation Management when learning of this step (Ascher et al. 2013).

The second step involves recognizing that a greater power can restore one's sanity. The second step has been a barrier for many people since it can seem to imply specific religious beliefs. While AA developed from within the Protestant religious tradition, AA has never endorsed a particular religion—the only requirement for membership is a desire to stop drinking (Alcoholics Anonymous 1956). References to a higher power often include the phrase, "as one understands him," and many nonreligious AA members link "higher power" with the power of the group—specifically believing that their sobriety is possible only through the active participation of the AA group. Nevertheless, some individuals prefer to attend programs that have omitted reference to a higher power; these include AA Beyond Belief and SMART recovery (Ascher et al. 2013).

Most people with CODs are able to work within the above 12-step structure as well as people with SUDs who lack an additional psychiatric diagnosis. Of course, meaningfully participating in a group requires a certain amount of impulse control and cognitive ability; some patients with mania and psychosis, for example, would likely be too agitated to work within a 12-step framework. As their most acute symptoms are controlled, many are able to successfully return to their 12-step program.

Historically, AA members have, at times, extended the philosophy of abstinence to include psychiatric medications (Meissen et al. 1999). This led some people with CODs to have to choose between their psychiatric medications and AA attendance. This requirement of complete medication abstinence is currently unusual—even the original Big Book specifically recommended that its members be able to make use of necessary psychiatric care, including medications. It should also be remembered that AA came into existence before the advent of haloperidol, chlorpromazine, and the tricyclic antidepressants. At present, people with CODs should be able to readily receive psychiatric care and participate in 12-step programs (Meissen et al. 1999).

As is generally true for any groups, AA groups can be intimidating to newcomers. AA anticipates this group process, and a core precept is that one's own recovery depends on helping other people maintain sobriety; this mandate leads more experienced members to proactively include newcomers, which can ease recovery in people whose anxiety or depression might otherwise preclude participation in a group.

Run by members rather than professionals, AA has succeeded for reasons that include minimal cost and wide-spread availability. Following the success of AA, there was extensive growth of 12-step programs for other addictive and problematic behaviors. These include Narcotics Anonymous, Marijuana Anonymous (MA), Cocaine Anonymous (CA), and Gamblers Anonymous (GA), among others. They share in common the 12 steps with minor variations.

We present a case of a man with substance use and a persistent, severe mental disorder. His situation is pertinent, especially since he is someone who profited from 12-step programs despite a severe, persistent mental illness that might have made him seem like an unlikely candidate for the program. The case presentation will focus on how the use of a 12-step program was a pivotal piece of the treatment of his CODs.

## Clinical Case

Manuel is a 45-year-old man who had originally presented to our outpatient psychiatric clinic 7 years earlier with persistent psychosis, chronic cocaine and alcohol use disorders, multiple prior psychiatric hospitalizations, and homelessness.

At the time of his initial presentation to the clinic, Manuel had been using alcohol and cocaine almost continuously for more than 20 years (since age 16). He had been first hospitalized psychiatrically for psychosis at age 18. At that time, he was diagnosed with substance-induced psychosis. Two years later, he was hospitalized for 3 months (the hospitalization was precipitated by a motor vehicle accident but prolonged for psychiatric reasons). At that time, it was noted that auditory hallucinations, ideas of reference, paranoia, and cognitive disorganization improved somewhat while Manuel was taking antipsychotic medication but that Manuel remained psychotic throughout his 12-week hospitalization. Because of that lengthy period of abstinence with persistent psychosis, his diagnosis was changed to schizophrenia. At that time, he was discharged on antipsychotic medications, which he promptly discontinued.

During the ensuing two decades, Manuel was periodically taken to emergency rooms by the police with a description of being an "emotionally disturbed person." His parents, who were both schoolteachers, tried to get their only child to take the prescribed medications but were unsuccessful. He often lived with them, but he would routinely disappear for weeks or months at a time. He tended to explain later that he had been forced to leave his parents because they were spying on him or trying to poison him. During his many ED visits, his urine toxicology was generally positive for cocaine, and his blood alcohol level tended to indicate intoxication.

Manuel's trials of antipsychotic medication tended to be incomplete, but they included haloperidol, risperidone, and olanzapine. During one psychiatric hospitalization, clozapine seemed to lead to the resolution of most of his positive symptoms, though he remained suspicious and isolated. To address his substance abuse, he attended at least three rehabilitation programs, though he never appeared to follow up after discharge, almost always relapsing on alcohol and cocaine upon discharge. After his father and then his mother died, he became persistently homeless and psychotic, using alcohol and cocaine as much as he could afford.

At the age of 38, Manuel was discharged from an acute psychiatric unit into a residence for the homeless mentally ill and chemically addicted (i.e., a MICA residence). As part of this program, he entered an outpatient dual diagnosis clinic. Manuel seemed to get traction with a program that combined many elements. Not only did the MICA residence provide housing and access to a psychiatrist and social worker, it also offered some degree of social acceptance and organization. With this structure, he could accept ongoing supportive psychotherapy and antipsychotic medications.

Manuel had been offered 12-step programs as part of his prior rehabilitations. In the context of persistent psychosis, psychosocial disruption, homelessness, and almost continuous substance abuse, Manuel had never found them helpful. After a period of enforced abstinence and while living in a MICA unit where he began to make some friends, Manuel finally got traction within the 12-step program. Manuel found his Double Trouble in Recovery (DTR) group to be especially effective. DTR is a 12-step program that has been adapted for people with CODs.[1] The first step has, for example, been adapted to read as follows: "We admitted we were powerless over our mental disorders and substance abuse—that our lives had become unmanageable." He began to go to a DTR meeting every morning and would often go to one more 12-step meeting later in the day. By obtaining social security disability and getting access to a small inheritance, Manuel was also able to find supportive housing. He developed a daily routine that included his morning DTR meeting; coffee and the newspaper; a walk through the park; a nap; a meeting or phone call with his sponsor; and supper with friends from the program. He appeared to be adherent to clozapine, which reduced his auditory hallucinations and paranoia. He attended individual psychotherapy sessions, which helped him develop coping strategies when he was feeling especially paranoid.

Manuel has had at least four psychotic relapses during the last 7 years. In each case, his sponsor recognized characteristic symptoms: being absent from daily DTR meetings, skipping their daily coffee or phone call, maintaining interpersonal silence, and having a "crazy look in his eye." In each case, the sponsor brought Manuel to the emergency room that is affiliated with Manuel's outpatient clinic. Each time, Manuel rebounded within a few days and was able to be released back to his apartment.

During his ongoing supportive psychotherapy, Manuel was limited by his persistent tendency toward suspiciousness and by some cognitive decline consistent with schizophrenia and persistent substance abuse. Nevertheless, he recalled being the only child born to immigrant parents. They had "done everything" for him, and his childhood was "perfect." He felt guilty that he repeatedly hurt and disappointed them. He sometimes felt terribly lonely and sad that they had died before he was able to make amends. At his DTR group, he takes special pride in helping out "guys from the streets, guys like me." And he believes that his parents can watch him as he shows up every morning, ready to help another of "his guys."

---

[1]Hazelden Foundation 1993.

# Discussion

Manuel has co-occurring schizophrenia and two SUDs (cocaine and alcohol). After decades of a downward spiral, he appears to have halted his slide and gained traction through a combination of treatments that include enforced abstinence, residence within a MICA program, adherence to antipsychotic medication, and his alliances with a psychotherapist and with an effective social worker. Manuel would probably say that his 12-step group was, by far, the key factor in his improvement, but it seems unlikely that any one intervention would have been effective without the others.

Manuel has a history that is fairly typical of someone who is recurrently identified by police and emergency rooms as an "emotionally disturbed person." He has a persistent, severe mental illness (schizophrenia). He is inadequately adherent to medications. He is often homeless. While Manuel has severe substance abuse, his paranoia and disruptive behavior at times may make it difficult for him to tolerate a typical 12 step meeting (Bogenschutz et al. 2006; Book et al. 2009). His mental illness would also make it less likely that mental health specialists would refer him for a 12-step program (Humphreys 1997). His odd behavior might also reduce the likelihood that he would be accepted by a 12-step meeting if he did try to attend. Though most contact persons within AA appear to have positive attitudes toward individuals with CODs, a majority also believe that specialized groups for those with CODs would be more helpful than mainstream AA (Meissen et al. 1999). Although there is some evidence that people with co-occurring psychosis attend 12-step meetings less regularly (Westermeyer and Schneekloth 1999), most studies have found that individuals with CODs attend 12-step groups at rates approaching those of others with SUDs (Bogenschutz et al. 2006).

Several studies have investigated the relationship of 12-step attendance and outcomes for individuals with CODs. Most of these studies focus on a population of Veterans Affairs (VA) patients, which limits generalizability. There is strong evidence of association between attendance in 12-step programs and clinical improvement in substance use symptoms. In addition, there is some evidence of improvement in psychiatric symptoms. However, it is unclear if individuals with CODs benefit from 12-step participation to the same extent as those with substance use disorders only (Bogenschutz et al. 2006). Some evidence shows higher rates of abstinence, better adherence to psychiatric medication, and improved personal functioning in those attending dual-focused groups rather than AA/NA (Magura et al. 2003; Timko 2008).

## PHARMACOLOGICAL INTERVENTIONS

It is not clear why Manuel did not take his antipsychotic medications for many years, but it seems to have had more to do with his paranoia than with potential stigma emanating from members of 12-step groups (which he generally did not attend during those years). Nevertheless, the clinician should be actively aware that some patients may be counseled to stop their psychiatric medications (including medications for their SUDs like buprenorphine, methadone, and naltrexone) as part of their abstinence program. It should also be recalled, however, that there is evidence that the more typical attitude within AA is that people with CODs should take their psychiatric medications (Meissen et al. 1999).

# Conclusion

Twelve-step programs are widely available and effective treatments for individuals with and without CODs. While patients may opt to not attend such programs for a number of reasons, clinicians and patients should be aware that psychiatric symptoms rarely result in someone not being able to participate in such groups. Further, there are even 12-step programs designed especially for individuals with CODs.

## KEY POINTS

- Twelve-step programs such as Alcoholics Anonymous (AA) and Narcotics Anonymous (NA) are effective.

- Psychiatric symptomatology may negatively affect participation in 12-step programs. The symptomatology can, however, generally be tolerated. In other cases, individuals benefit from attendance at programs tailored to those with co-occurring disorders.

- Double Trouble in Recovery is a specialized mutual-help program designed by and for the dually diagnosed to create a more welcoming environment tailored to this community.

- Twelve-step participation rates for individuals with co-occurring disorders are generally comparable to those for individuals with substance use disorders without co-occurring conditions.

# Questions

1. How many members does Alcoholics Anonymous (AA) have?

    A. 100,000.
    B. 500,000.
    C. 1 million.
    D. 2 million+.

2. Which of the following is *true* about AA or Narcotics Anonymous (NA)?

    A. AA was the first mutual aid fellowship to encourage abstinence from alcohol in its members.
    B. A belief in God is an essential component of NA.
    C. Most 12-step programs discourage members from taking psychiatric medications.
    D. The only requirement for AA membership is a desire to stop drinking.

3. Which of the following is *true* regarding 12-step participation and individuals with co-occurring disorders (CODs)?

    A. Twelve-step participation rates in individuals with CODs are generally comparable to those in individuals with substance use disorders (SUDs) only.
    B. Individuals with CODs are more likely to be referred to 12-step programs than are those with SUDs only.
    C. Individuals with CODs attending Double Trouble in Recovery (DTR) have lower rates of abstinence than individuals attending AA with substance use disorders only.
    D. A major disadvantage of 12-step programs is cost.

# References

Alcoholics Anonymous: A.A. Fact file. 1956. Available at: http://www.aa.org/assets/en_US/m-24_aafactfile.pdf. Accessed February 7, 2017.

Alcoholics Anonymous: Alcoholics Anonymous: Twelve Steps and Twelve Traditions. New York, Alcoholics Anonymous World Services, 1978

Ascher M, Wittenauer J, Avery J: Alternatives to the 12-step groups. Curr Psychiatr 12(9):E1–E2, 2013

Bogenschutz MP, Geppert CM, George J: The role of twelve-step approaches in dual diagnosis treatment and recovery. Am J Addict 15(1):50–60, 2006 16449093

Book SW, Thomas SE, Dempsey JP, et al: Social anxiety impacts willingness to participate in addiction treatment. Addict Behav 34(5):474–476, 2009 19195794

Hazelden Foundation: Double Trouble in Recovery. Center City, MN, Hazelden Foundation, 1993

Humphreys K: Clinicians' referral and matching of substance abuse patients to self-help groups after treatment. Psychiatr Serv 48(11):1445–1449, 1997 9355173

Magura S, Laudet AB, Mahmood D, et al: Role of self-help processes in achieving abstinence among dually diagnosed persons. Addict Behav 28(3):399–413, 2003 12628615

Meissen G, Powell TJ, Wituk SA, et al: Attitudes of AA contact persons toward group participation by persons with a mental illness. Psychiatr Serv 50(8):1079–1081, 1999 10445659

Nace EP: Twelve-step programs in addiction recovery, in The ASAM Principles of Addiction Medicine, 5th Edition. Edited by Ries R, Fiellin DA, Miller SC, Saitz R, et al. Philadelphia, PA, Lippincott Williams & Wilkins, 2014, pp 1033–1042

Timko C: Outcomes of AA for special populations. Recent Dev Alcohol 18:373–392, 2008 19115780

Westermeyer JJ, Schneekloth TD: Course of substance abuse in patients with and without schizophrenia. Am J Addict 8(1):55–64, 1999 10189515

# 12

# MOTIVATIONAL INTERVIEWING

*Howard R. Steinberg, Ph.D.*
*David T. Pilkey, Ph.D.*
*Steve Martino, Ph.D.*

All psychotherapeutic treatments aim to help clients to make changes to improve their lives. Helping clients who have had enduring struggles with substance use and severe mental illness become motivated to make these changes may be daunting for many therapists. Therapists might feel considerable pressure to immediately intervene with prescribed medications, intensive case management services, and various efforts to develop clients' coping skills and personal resources. The challenge occurs when these clients are not ready to commit to such treatment interventions and continue to approach their problems in unproductive and sometimes self-destructive ways.

Over the past two decades, motivation enhancement has become the focus of treatment for people with co-occurring disorders (CODs). These approaches typically aim to engage clients in treatment and, thereby, improve treatment outcomes (Hettema et al. 2005; Lundahl et al. 2010; Smedslund et al. 2011; Zuckoff and Daley 2001). The most widely utilized and studied among these motivational therapies, particularly for the treatment of substance use problems, is *motivational interviewing* (MI). MI is described by Miller and Rollnick as "a person-centered counseling style for addressing the common problem of ambivalence about change" (Miller and Rollnick 2013, p. 21). In MI, therapists engage their clients in a conversation that serves to increase clients' intrinsic motivation for change. Using a highly empathic and supportive interviewing style, therapists attempt to understand their clients' perceptions of their problems and help them resolve ambivalence toward making changes.

Miller and Rollnick have identified four overlapping processes of MI: engaging, focusing, evoking, and planning (Table 12–1) (Miller and Rollnick 2013). In *engaging*, therapists work to establish a good working relationship with their clients and learn how their clients view their presenting problems. *Focusing* is the process by which clients and therapists agree on the change target. Drawing out clients' motivations for changing targeted behaviors is the process referred to as *evoking*, with the aim of preparing clients to make a commitment to change. Finally, *planning* involves strengthening commitment to change by developing a plan that specifies steps and supports or resources clients will use to enact change.

To effectively implement the processes to help bring about change, MI therapists ask questions that conform to the acronym OARS. The questions are *open-ended* and *affirm* positive aspects of their clients. The clinicians use *reflective* listening and provide balanced *summaries* of what their clients have presented during the interview. Additionally, therapists consistently look to promote their clients' expression of arguments that favor change, which is referred to as "change talk" within MI.

Additional MI therapeutic techniques include asking questions that draw out clients' *desire, ability, reasons,* and *need* (DARN) to change (Table 12–2). In addition, assuming clients indicate a *commitment* to make a change, therapists may further *activate* this commitment by determining what their clients might be willing to do to prepare for change and then examine how clients might begin to *take steps* (CAT) toward change. As therapists guide their clients to express arguments for change and diminish those against it (i.e., sustain talk), the clients quite literally talk themselves into change based on their own self-motivations.

When using MI, therapists interact with their clients with *MI spirit.* MI spirit has four key elements that conform to the acronym PACE: partnership, acceptance, compassion, and evocation. *Partnership* means that therapists understand, respect, and value their clients' perspective

**TABLE 12–1.** The four processes of motivational interviewing

| Process | Description |
|---------|-------------|
| Engaging | Establishing a good working relationship and learning about the client |
| Focusing | Agreeing on the target of motivational enhancement and directing the conversation toward it |
| Evoking | Drawing out the client's own motivations for changing the target behavior to prepare the client to commit to change |
| Planning | Strengthening commitment to change through the formulation of a specific plan of action |

and autonomy. It presumes a collaborative working relationship throughout treatment. *Acceptance* indicates that therapists value their clients as human beings, respect their rights and abilities to make their own choices, and search for and recognize their clients' strengths and efforts. Therapists meet their clients where they are motivationally without judgment. *Compassion* means therapists seek what is in the best interest of their clients rather than promoting change that primarily would benefit others. Hence, therapists do not use MI in situations in which the best interests of their clients are not clear (e.g., making a decision about organ donation). *Evocation* requires that therapists believe that the potential for change exists in their clients. This stance is critical in MI in that it forms the basis for therapists to draw out their clients' thoughts and values that support change and limits the chance that therapists will impose their own arguments for clients to change.

In this chapter we describe the use of MI with an individual who suffers from CODs. We provide a discussion of the case that includes the interplay of substance use and psychiatric and psychosocial issues, and describe how we used MI to help the client enhance his motivation to change. We conclude the case presentation with a discussion of clinical considerations in the use of MI with clients who have dual substance use and psychiatric disorders.

## Clinical Case

John is a 42-year-old, divorced Army veteran who is being evaluated within the Veterans Administration (VA) health care system. John describes at least 7 years of recurrent alcohol binges.

**TABLE 12–2. Examples of evocative questions that evoke change talk: DARN-CAT**

| Change talk category | Therapist evocative question | Client change talk response |
|---|---|---|
| Desire | What would you like to be different? | I'd like more money in my pocket. |
| Ability | What has helped you not use crack in the past? | I went to a residential program to get away from all the people, places, and things causing me trouble. |
| Reason | What are the advantages of not smoking cigarettes? | If I quit smoking, I'd be a better example for my kids. |
| Need | How urgent is not drinking right now? | It's really urgent. I caught my daughter being drunk and I have no credibility to tell her not to drink and certainly not to get drunk. |
| Commitment | Given what we have discussed, what would you like to do? | I'm going to try that medication. |
| Activation | What steps are you willing to take between now and your next appointment? | I am willing to go to a Narcotics Anonymous meeting held at the church around the corner Wednesday night. |
| Taking steps | How are you already moving in this direction? | I dumped out all the liquor I had in my house. |

He has been repeatedly arrested and psychiatrically hospitalized. He is unemployed, socially isolated, financially strained, and divorced from his wife of 17 years due in great part to his drinking.

John reports that his drinking gradually escalated during his 20 years of military service. Since John has returned to civilian life, his drinking has increased to a pint of vodka per day with regular binges. He has been arrested twice for driving under the influence. He has been charged with disorderly conduct at least four times for bar fights. By John's report and according to VA records, he appears to have had six prior alcohol treatments, including five medically assisted detoxifications. These treatments have become steadily more complicated.

Eight months prior to this presentation, John was admitted for another detox, followed by participation in an intensive outpatient program. Throughout that treatment, John's speech was pressured, and he displayed insomnia, paranoia, grandiosity, irritability, and a tendency to being easily triggered into violence. His symptoms were most consistent with bipolar disorder, consistent with his family history.

John has had a rocky treatment trajectory. He had been initially enthusiastic about working with the intensive outpatient treatment staff, but he had become frustrated by the adverse side effects of his mood-stabilizing medications. Though he managed to not drink alcohol for a few days at a time, John was arrested again for alcohol-fueled fights. He was discharged from the program, though he later contacted program staff members who encouraged John to reengage in treatment.

John presents at this time for a combined residential and intensive outpatient treatment program that consists of cognitive-behavioral therapy, motivational interviewing, and 12-step facilitation in a group format. Additionally, veterans receive case management services from residential treatment program staff.

## Discussion

We organize our discussion of John's treatment according to the four main MI processes: engaging, focusing, evoking, and planning. We demonstrate components of MI with each process and how we systematically worked with John to enhance his motivation and resolve his ambivalence toward change, consistent with the spirit of the approach. For each process, we provide dialogue to illustrate MI in practice.

## ENGAGING

Establishing a strong working relationship is essential to MI, a process that may be especially challenging when working with individuals with CODs. Engagement can be enhanced by using the OARS techniques (Open ended, Affirmative, Reflective, Summarizing). Program therapists used open-ended questions to explore John's condition, concerns, and reasons for coming into treatment. In addition, the therapists looked for opportunities to affirm John's strengths and any steps he had taken toward change as a means to build rapport and simultaneously begin to promote his self-efficacy. Finally, the therapists used summaries to place John's statements within a broader picture and to bring added emphasis to his change talk. The following dialogue is an example of the engagement process with John:

> THERAPIST: What brings you to the program? (*open question inviting a client-centered problem discussion*)
> CLIENT: I've been through all of this before. I'm not really sure why I'm here again, but I guess I must be doing something wrong, and now I'm back in the program and will have to listen to everyone's stories again.
> THERAPIST: You're concerned that you've been doing something wrong. (*reflection*)
> CLIENT: Well, yeah. If I was doing the right thing, then I wouldn't have ended up in the hospital, I wouldn't have been arrested again, and I wouldn't be here.
> THERAPIST: You don't want to be here, and you think some of the things you've been doing have led you to be here now. (*reflection*)
> CLIENT: They say it was because I went off of my meds. I don't really think that's it, but that's what they're telling me. I really hate taking them. I just ended up getting carried away with the drinking again. That's all this is really about.
> THERAPIST: You're not happy about taking your medications; however, it was your drinking that led you back into the hospital again and ultimately here. Tell me more about the drinking. (*reflection with open question*)
> CLIENT: The drinking always gets me in trouble. I end up getting depressed, or really pissed off, and then I drink and end up in the hospital, or worse, getting arrested for something stupid. I'm tired of it.
> THERAPIST: You don't want this cycle to continue over and over again. Even though you really don't want to be here again, you've had enough of what the drinking has been doing to your life, like in-

terfering with taking your meds and, worse yet, getting into legal problems and being hospitalized over and over again. You're looking for a way to make some type of change in how things have been going for you. (*summary*)

CLIENT: I have to do something. I don't want to end up in jail again. I just want to be able to get by like other people and sometimes that includes not wanting to take meds for my Bipolar. Maybe there is something this time around that will help. I don't know.

THERAPIST: You want to do something different to make a change in your life. Despite not being thrilled to be here, you're considering making good use of this program. I can hear your willingness to take a look at the cycle you keep getting caught in and maybe even learn how to approach things differently. (*affirmation*)

## FOCUSING

When working with individuals with CODs, it can be difficult for the therapist and client to agree on targets for motivational enhancement. There may be multiple problem behaviors operating at the same time, which may overwhelm both client and therapist. The process of focusing requires that the therapist works with the client to identify potential areas for motivational enhancement and to prioritize them such that there is a clear direction during the interview. Moreover, the client may present with significant ambivalence about changing an area very relevant to his or her recovery (e.g., drinking, medication and treatment adherence). Focusing requires that the therapist and client come together to work on an agreed-upon issue, which may require some negotiation. The following is an example of how the therapist might handle the process of bringing focus to the interview with John:

CLIENT: I know I have to do something, but it seems like every time I try to make a change, I end up back in the same place. It seems like too much to deal with now.

THERAPIST: You're worried that if you put in the effort to make some changes in your life now, that it may not work out; that it may be a waste of your time.

CLIENT: Well, it probably won't be a complete waste of time, but I just don't want to feel like a failure again.

THERAPIST: I can understand that. I agree with you that if you're going to decide and make some changes in your life, it's important to find a way to be able to see some real changes happen. You had mentioned having a number of problems that you needed to deal with. Do you think it would be helpful for you if we focused on one problem at a time?

CLIENT: Maybe. I'm not really sure where to start though. They keep wanting me to take my meds, but I'm just not sure about that.

THERAPIST: So, maybe starting somewhere other than the medications may be better right now. You had mentioned drinking sometimes gets you into trouble.

CLIENT: That's an understatement.

THERAPIST: You told me that when you're drinking too much, that it leads to some other problems, including problems with your mood, and even some legal problems.

CLIENT: Yeah. This has gone on too long.

THERAPIST: Do you think that this would be a good place to start?

CLIENT: I guess so. I'm not sure that I can stop drinking forever, but I know that I need to do something about it.

## EVOKING

Once treatment focus has been established and the client remains engaged in the conversation, the therapist prioritizes drawing out and bringing emphasis to the client's change talk. The client's psychiatric condition can complicate the interview. For example, active psychiatric symptoms, unwanted effects of prescribed medications, and cognitive limitations may impede motivational enhancement (Martino et al. 2002). Nonetheless, a key issue in evoking change talk is the therapist's capacity to recognize the client's change talk when it occurs.

It is useful for the therapist to engage with the client while attending to change talk as summarized by the acronym DARN-CAT (desire, ability, reasons, and need—commitment, activation, and taking steps). When motives are spontaneously articulated, the therapist typically asks the client to elaborate more about them. In addition, the therapist might use a variety of strategies to deliberately evoke change talk and resolve ambivalence toward change. Asking open questions that pull for this information is often the best way to go about encouraging the client to discuss change (see Table 12–2). Some common evocative questions include "What might you do to make a change?" "What are some reasons why you might want to make a change?" and "What are some of the advantages of making this change?"

When change talk occurs, the therapist responds to these statements in ways that encourage similar talk. Miller and Rollnick (2013) suggest that therapists ask for examples or elaboration on the change talk provided. Reflections, affirmations, and summaries may also provide the client opportunities to further explore and expand upon the change talk being offered. Other commonly used strategies (Table 12–3) include using scaling rulers, exploring goals or values, asking the client to look forward or back in time, and exploring strengths or past successes to help improve the client's sense of change efficacy. The following interview with John contains several evocative elements:

THERAPIST: Tell me a little more about your thoughts on the medication you have been prescribed. When you brought it up before, you looked pretty frustrated.

CLIENT: You know, I am frustrated…I'd say angry is more like it. Each time I take it, they can't seem to get the right dose, and I end up feeling like a zombie. I can't get anything done when I feel that way, so I stop taking it. No wonder why I end up drinking.

THERAPIST: You're trying to take what is prescribed for you, but instead of helping, you feel like it is making things worse. (*reflection of implied effort to take medication*)

CLIENT: Exactly! Now you can see why I drink. Alcohol helps me calm down and feel better…something the medication should be doing. I don't want to keep messing up and getting drunk all the time, but I don't know what else to do.

THERAPIST: There's an important connection. If I am hearing you right, you recognize the meds might be necessary for your mood, but the ones you're taking now aren't working well enough and will need to be changed or adjusted. If you can get your meds in better order, you think you would be far less likely to drink. (*reflection of benefits of mood-stabilizing medications*)

CLIENT: Yeah. That's exactly what I'm saying.

THERAPIST: And you feel you could stop drinking if the medications helped you with your mood without giving you the bad side effects. (*reflection of ability to not drink under certain conditions*)

CLIENT: Sure. I mean I'm pretty sure I could, though I don't have a very good track record.

THERAPIST: So, the only way you could imagine yourself not drinking is if your meds get fixed. (*amplified reflection of sustain talk to reveal the change talk side of ambivalence*)

CLIENT: Well, I know that I should stop drinking. I really need to stop. If I get arrested again I won't be able to get a job. I'll lose everything. I don't want that to happen.

THERAPIST: It sounds like staying sober is really important to you. If I hear you correctly, you would be able to work again and maybe things would start getting back on track for you. (*reflection of cons of continued drinking*)

CLIENT: I hope so. You know I did pretty well when I was in the Army. When I put my mind to something, I know I can get it done.

THERAPIST: I believe you can. What do you think you might be able to do in the next few days that would help you to maintain better control of your mood and to make it more likely for you to stay sober? (*affirmation of strengths followed by evocative question*)

CLIENT: Well, people keep talking about how I need to take my medication, but I only want to take it if it will really help me. I'm just confused. Can you guarantee that my meds will help?

**TABLE 12–3. Other evocative strategies**

| | |
|---|---|
| Using scaling rulers | An importance ruler uses a scale (0–10) to determine level of perceived importance of change.<br><br>A confidence ruler uses a scale (0–10) to determine perceived confidence in carrying out the change.<br><br>For each ruler, once the client selects a number, the therapist asks why not a lower number (i.e., "Why a 4 and not a 1?") to elicit change talk. The therapist can then ask what would increase importance or confidence (i.e., "What would help that number go from a 4 to a 5?") to elicit further change talk. |
| Exploring or reflecting pros for change and cons for no change | The therapist explores or reflects the client's arguments that would support change, namely, the pros or benefits of implementing a behavioral change and the cons or drawbacks of not making a change. Often referred to as a *decisional balance*, in MI this strategy does not give equal emphasis to the arguments against change (pros for not changing and cons for changing). Rather, the emphasis is placed on the elicitation of change talk rather than a neutral exploration of all sides of the change issue under consideration. |
| Exploring goals and values | The therapist explores a client's important goals or values and then asks the patient how they fit with his or her current behavior, which may develop discrepancy and create motivation for change. The therapist also asks how the client's goals or values would be affected if change were to occur. |
| Looking forward, back, or at extremes | The therapist asks the client to look forward into the future and imagine how the client's life would improve if change were to occur. The therapist also could ask the client to look back in time to a period of healthier functioning and contrast it with current circumstances. |

**TABLE 12–3.   Other evocative strategies** (*continued*)

| | |
|---|---|
| Exploring strengths or past successes | The therapist explores the client's strengths and past successes and asks the client to consider how these strengths or skills used to achieve success might apply to current circumstances. This discussion might improve the client's sense of ability to change. |
| Exchanging information | The therapist provides information with the client's permission (either by asking for it or when the therapist is asked) in a way that emphasizes the client's autonomy. The therapist asks what the client makes of the shared information. The therapist might use another strategy called "elicit-provide-elicit." Here, the therapist first explores what the client knows about a subject, then provides additional or corrective information, and concludes by asking how the client received the information. |

THERAPIST: You want to be sure that if you're going to give the medication a try that you'll end up feeling better and then, staying sober will be easier for you. It also sounds as if you may need some more information about your medications. Would you mind if I made a suggestion? (*reflection of ability to not drink under certain conditions, asking permission to exchange information*)

CLIENT: Go ahead.

THERAPIST: You might consider having an open conversation with your psychiatrist about your medications. You can ask her about different side effects, you can go over medication options, and you can express to her what you and I talked about, namely, that you're interested in getting help with your mood so that you can have a better shot at staying sober. What do you think? (*exchanging information and eliciting the client's response*)

CLIENT: I don't really want to, but I was just telling you that I have to do something. I think I can do that.

THERAPIST: This is clearly very important to you. What do you think about making an appointment with her? (*reflection emphasizing the importance of the client's goal and asking for a commitment*)

CLIENT: I'll call her today.

## PLANNING

In the planning process of MI, we are essentially asking the client, "So, what comes next?" If the client expresses a willingness to make a change, then it is appropriate to work with the client to put a plan together, or perhaps, the first steps in an initial plan that will be revisited and revised as the client attempts change over time. Overall, planning entails setting a targeted change goal, having the client describe steps to take to make the change, identifying social supports, anticipating potential obstacles and how to address them, and asking the client to reaffirm commitment to the plan.

When working with individuals who experience chronic substance use and psychiatric problems, ambivalence about change may rise to the surface again during the change planning process. This experience is normal and natural at the point in which someone is making a commitment, much like the "cold feet" phenomenon before marriage (Miller and Rollnick 2013). Attempting to push through this ambivalence in an effort to get the client to commit to an agreed-upon plan likely will backfire in that the client will argue the side of no change to counterbalance the therapist's statements. Instead, patiently reflecting this expected ambivalence may help the client to revisit reasons for change and allow for the continuation of the change planning process.

In the prior dialogue, John committed to contacting his psychiatrist to discuss his medications. In the next example, John and his therapist develop a change plan and work through his temporary hesitation involving his fear that the medications will continue to be bothersome:

THERAPIST: I've heard you describe some concerns about your drinking and how your mood can trigger you to drink. You're not opposed to taking mood-stabilizing medication. You just want them to have fewer side effects. Having that meeting with your psychiatrist may help her understand what some of your difficulties have been. You said you plan to call her to discuss this issue.

CLIENT: Well, I really don't think it will help. I mean, I know I have to stop the drinking, but what are the chances that she can get the meds to work the right way for me? I doubt it is going to be worth it.

THERAPIST: You know that it's really important to change your drinking behavior, and getting the medications right is part of the plan to reach that goal. At the same time, you doubt meeting with her to discuss your medications will be helpful. (*reflecting client's ambivalence about medication adherence*)

CLIENT: Right. I don't know. I just hate the idea that I may be setting myself up for another failure.

THERAPIST: Because setting yourself up for failure may affect your mood, and you're concerned this may lead you to drink—something you said you don't want to do. (*reflecting the client's goal to not drink*)

CLIENT: Maybe. I really hate the side effects of the medication. If it wasn't for that, I don't think I would have such a problem with taking them. I know I don't usually drink when I'm taking them.

THERAPIST: This isn't easy for you. You identified that you need to do something about the drinking, and that you don't typically drink when you take your medications. However, the side effects can be tough to deal with. (*reflecting client's ambivalence about medication adherence*)

CLIENT: I already told you the drinking has to stop, and if there's a chance that speaking with my psychiatrist about the problems with the medication may help, then I can at least talk to her about it.

THERAPIST: From what you have told me so far, how do you want to proceed? (*supporting the client's autonomy*)

CLIENT: I need to make that call. I'll call her today to make the appointment.

# Conclusion

John's case shows how severe mental illness and substance use disorders interact with each other to complicate the motivational enhancement process for treatment adherence and targeted behavior change. When working with John, the therapist addressed several behavioral targets (mania, medication adherence, drinking) during the course of the interview. However, the therapist primarily focused on where the client wanted to concentrate his change effort (drinking) and then considered with the client how his mood instability and use of medications interacted with his drinking. The therapist then recognized, reinforced, and elicited change talk about not drinking, including change talk about medication adherence and improved mood stability in the service of reaching his alcohol abstinence goal.

Because John had sufficient psychiatric stability at the time of the motivational interviews, using MI was warranted. The use of MI when a client's symptom severity hampers the client's capacity to respond to the treatment's processes becomes more challenging. Clients may have difficulty accurately appraising the consequences of problematic behaviors or maintaining a logical course of conversation. In addition, they may misinterpret the meaning of statements and comments by the therapist because of symptoms of their primary psychiatric illness; psychosis, depression, and mania can all impact on the client's ability to attend to the therapist and engage in self-reflection. Although MI may not be useful with certain clients some of the time, even the most severely impaired patients can benefit from tactful variations of MI and the MI spirit.

Martino and Moyers have provided specific suggestions for modifying MI when working with individuals with CODs (Martino and Moyers 2008). They emphasize open-ended and evocative questions to elicit a discussion of the interaction between the individual's psychiatric condition and his or her substance use problem. They also describe the importance of a focus on adherence to both medication and treatment programs, as well as attending to the motivation to use substances. Finally, they suggest using clear and concise terms, successively reflecting and summarizing frequently, and using more engaging and concrete methods to elicit change talk. Utilizing these skills also provides the opportunity to collect a running assessment of the client's mental status and helps keep the client organized.

In most cases, MI alone is insufficient to treat individuals with CODs. Over the course of the interview, John's motivation for changing his drinking and addressing his medication adherence issues were drawn out into the open. A specific plan to not drink hinged in part on his working out an improved mood stabilizing medication regimen with fewer adverse effects. However, the development of specific coping skills, social skills training, other psychosocial interventions, pharmacological interventions, and emotion regulation strategies are often important components of comprehensive treatment for individuals with complex presentations, and these interventions are not a part of MI. Additionally, MI may not be the appropriate strategy to use during a crisis or in the midst of a transfer between institutions. Nevertheless, the techniques and spirit of MI can be helpful in a wide variety of difficult situations.

## KEY POINTS

- Motivational interviewing (MI) is an evidence-based treatment in which the therapist helps the client resolve ambivalence about a change in an effort to enhance the client's intrinsic motivation and commitment to change.

- When using MI with individuals who have co-occurring disorders, the therapist must make every effort to engage the client in the interview, identify a specific problem focus for motivational enhancement, identify and evoke change talk, and resolve ambivalence toward change prior to moving forward with developing plans for change.

- Individuals with comorbid substance use disorders and severe mental illness may bring unique challenges to the delivery of MI. Such challenges may be directly tied to the acuity of the psychiatric disorder; to the recency, severity, and type of substance use; and to the pressing psychosocial stressors experienced by the client.

# Questions

1. The first process in motivational interviewing (MI) is

    A. Assessment.
    B. Screening.
    C. Engaging.
    D. Planning.

2. The specific problem focus of MI treatment is determined by which of the following?

    A. Therapist.
    B. Client.
    C. Referral source.
    D. Client's past history.

3. Which of the following should be avoided when using MI with individuals with co-occurring disorders?

    A. Targeting medication and treatment program adherence in addition to substance use.

    B. Using successive reflections and summaries.

    C. Incorporating concrete and engaging methods for eliciting change talk.

    D. Discussing complex psychodynamic formulations.

# References

Hettema J, Steele J, Miller WR: Motivational interviewing. Annu Rev Clin Psychol 1:91–111, 2005 17716083

Lundahl B, Kunz C, Brownell C, et al: A meta-analysis of motivational interviewing: Twenty five years of empirical studies. Res Soc Work Pract 20:137–160, 2010

Martino S, Moyers TB: Motivational interviewing with dually diagnosed patients, in Motivational Interviewing in the Treatment of Psychological Problems. Edited by Arkowitz H, Westra HA, Miller WR, Rollnick S. New York, Guilford, 2008, pp 277–303

Martino S, Carroll K, Kostas D, et al: Dual Diagnosis Motivational Interviewing: a modification of Motivational Interviewing for substance-abusing patients with psychotic disorders. J Subst Abuse Treat 23(4):297–308, 2002 12495791

Miller WR, Rollnick S: Motivational Interviewing: Helping People Change, 3rd Edition. New York, Guilford, 2013

Smedslund G, Berg RC, Hammerstrøm KT, et al: Motivational interviewing for substance abuse. Cochrane Database Syst Rev 11(5):CD008063, 2011 21563163

Zuckoff A, Daley DC: Engagement and adherence issues in treating persons with nonpsychosis dual disorders. Psychiatr Rehabil Skills 5:131–162, 2001

# 13

# INPATIENT TREATMENT OF CO-OCCURRING DISORDERS

*Zain Khalid, M.D.*

*Sonal Batra, M.D.*

*Erin Zerbo, M.D.*

About half of the patients who are admitted for substance abuse treatment have a co-occurring psychiatric disorder (COD) (Center for Behavioral Health Statistics and Quality 2015). Within this large number of inpatient treatments is considerable heterogeneity. Not only do patients' specific substance use and psychiatric disorders vary, but so also do the severity of the CODs, the treatment histories, and the extent to which psychosocial factors impact on functioning. The mental health system is, itself, full of complexities that include local preferences, the availability of resources, and a multitude of potential treatments.

Although there is no definitive evidence for a specific cluster of interventions for any particular patient, there is a current set of best practices that can be applied to most patients who are admitted with CODs. In this chapter, we present the case of a man who was admitted to an inpatient unit for treatment of suicidality, depression, and three substance use disorders (SUDs) (opioids, alcohol, and tobacco). We then discuss admission criteria as well as the sorts of treatments that appear to be useful for this patient.

## Clinical Case

Dr. Kamin is a 34-year-old pharmacist who was brought to the emergency room by Emergency Medical Services (EMS). Dr. Kamin reported that he had been depressed and suicidal for months and had created his own "suicide stash" based on careful Internet review and his own knowledge of pharmaceuticals. After staring at his stash and drinking vodka for an hour, he had impulsively called 911. He regretted the phone call almost immediately, especially when he realized that not only would he be going to an emergency room, but that someone would confiscate his "only way out of this mess."

Dr. Kamin said that he had always been a "depressive guy," which had contributed to his "failure to meet women and have a normal life." About 3 years earlier, he had been injured in a motor vehicle accident, which led to a prescription of hydrocodone. The opioid was "transformative," and Dr. Kamin said he felt better with opioids than at any other time in his life. He described that he became more outgoing, more able to date, and had enjoyed weekends for the first time. When his pain physician would no longer prescribe opioids, he began stealing from the pharmacy where he worked. After a few months, the owner of the store confronted him about the theft. Dr. Kamin denied the allegation, fled the store, and never returned. He assumed that the owner never reported his suspicions about the theft, but he had been waiting for a visit from police for over a year. Dr. Kamin never went back to work as a pharmacist but instead lived off savings, which were about to run out.

While unemployed, Dr. Kamin bought oxycodone off the street, but he switched to heroin since it was cheaper. His maximum use had been up to 20 intranasal bags per day. He denied all intravenous use. He had also begun drinking more heavily. He said he typically drank about a pint of vodka daily, with greater amounts when opioids were hard to get and when he needed to function socially. He had tremors in the morning but had never had a withdrawal seizure or a medical admission for alcohol withdrawal. He had smoked 1 pack of cigarettes per day for the last 10 years. He denied the use of cocaine, marijuana, and other illicit substances.

About 1 year ago, his parents had "surprised [him] with an intervention." They had said that they were tired of watching him nod off at dinner whenever he let them into his apartment. Dr. Kamin had gone to a 28-day rehab, where he was introduced to "a bunch of the 12-step stuff." After finishing the rehab, he felt like he was on the proverbial "pink cloud" for several weeks but had then become increasingly demoralized, worried, and preoccupied about his future. During his 5 months of abstinence, he had not attended a therapy session or 12-step meeting, saying he figured he could do it by himself and noting that he wasn't a "group person." In regard to his relapse, he says that he spontaneously decided to let himself have one beer for his birthday, and, within an hour, he was buying heroin from his usual dealer. The pattern of his heroin and alcohol use quickly surpassed his previous pattern, and he simply could see no way out. He decided his "career was over." He felt alienated from his friends, sisters, and parents. He began to accumulate his "suicide stash" weeks earlier and was disappointed that he "lacked the guts" to get the job done.

Dr. Kamin is the youngest of three children born to a middle-class suburban family. He says that prior to his opioid use, his only vice has been a pack of cigarettes per day. Aside from his earlier rehab, he has never seen a mental health practitioner. He has never been married and has no children. His family history is significant only for parents who "worry all the time."

# Discussion

The evaluation of Dr. Kamin begins with a suicide assessment. He had carefully researched suicide, accumulated an apparently lethal number of pills, had seriously considered taking his "suicide stash" while intoxicated, and was disappointed that he had "lacked the guts" to follow through. He will need a psychiatric admission.

A second safety issue is whether he is likely to go into withdrawal from the alcohol. It appears that he has previously had only mild alcohol withdrawal, but the intensity of alcohol withdrawal can be difficult to predict, especially when the extent of alcohol use is often uncertain. Although less lethal than alcohol withdrawal, heroin and nicotine withdrawal can be very uncomfortable and lead to a difficult inpatient experience and the desire for a premature discharge.

A third important consideration is the exact differential diagnosis. It is clear that Dr. Kamin has alcohol, opioid, and tobacco use disorders.

Depressive symptoms appear to have precipitated the suicidality, though it is not completely clear whether the depression is primary or secondary to the use of heroin and alcohol. While the word "anxiety" is not specifically mentioned in the case, there are also hints that Dr. Kamin also has an undiagnosed anxiety disorder: his initial opioid use helped him be more sociable after a lifetime of being "unable to meet women." He is described as worried and preoccupied during his period of sobriety and to not be a "group person." He indicates that his parents are both worriers, as well, which hints at a family history of an anxiety disorder. Dr. Kamin may, therefore, have a primary anxiety and depressive disorder as well as the SUDs.

The presence of a co-occurring SUD, as in Dr. Kamin's case, appears to independently predict hospitalization even if the primary psychiatric illness is not very severe. CODs result in higher rates of hospitalization (Oh Min et al. 2005), higher treatment costs (Dickey and Azeni 1996), and higher rates of relapse and re-hospitalization (Haywood et al. 1995). Given these realities, it becomes crucial to make use of the best available evidence to develop effective treatment plans within the most appropriate setting.

While it may be fairly clear that Dr. Kamin needs an admission, the exact type of inpatient program may be less obvious. To address the complexity of CODs, guidelines have been proposed to create a "taxonomy" of addiction treatment programs (Mee-Lee et al. 2001). Treatment programs can be divided into three types: addiction-only services (AOS), dual diagnosis capable (DDC), and dual diagnosis enhanced (DDE). Psychiatric inpatient units tend to be DDE units, because a SUD without a co-occurring psychiatric diagnosis does not generally warrant a psychiatric admission. The taxonomy is based on a scoring system that takes into account multiple clinical variables, including acute intoxication and/or withdrawal potential; biomedical conditions and complications; emotional, behavioral, or cognitive conditions and complications; readiness to change; and the potential for relapse, continued use, or continued problems.

AOS programs focus entirely on people with SUDs and are unsuitable for people with prominent psychiatric symptoms. DDC programs focus primarily on persons with substance-related disorders but are also able to treat persons with less severe and/or more stable co-occurring psychiatric disorders. DDE programs are the most medically intensive and are capable of treating persons with more severe and debilitating mental illnesses as well as co-occurring substance-related disorders. Outcome data support the use of these criteria (Sharon et al. 2003; Stallvik and Gastfriend 2014).

The Patient Placement Criteria developed by the American Society of Addiction Medicine (ASAM) (Mee-Lee et al. 2001) offer one of the most comprehensive and useful guidelines for matching patients to appropriate treatment settings. Table 13–1 shows how the ASAM criteria could be applied to Dr. Kamin's case. Given the high severity of Dr. Kamin's co-occurring mental illness as assessed in Dimension 3, including the risk for self-harm and the combination of risks assessed in Dimensions 1, 2, 5, and 6, it is reasonable to initiate treatment at Level IV, a medically managed intensive inpatient, DDE service—otherwise known as a "dual diagnosis inpatient unit."

# Treatment

People with CODs fare better on units that focus on both conditions. It has been known for many years that parallel but separate services for SUDs and psychiatric illness have been shown to lead to service fragmentation, poor treatment adherence, and high dropout rates (Ridgely et al. 1990). In contrast, evidence indicates that coordinated inpatient programs that provide an integrated approach have better outcomes (Brunette et al. 2004). Further, programs that administer coordinated services sequentially (i.e., from inpatient treatment to residential rehabilitative facility) also have better outcomes (Moos et al. 2000). In regard to Dr. Kamin, he appears to have achieved a level of abstinence after his month-long rehab, but his recovery floundered in the context of inattention: neither he nor his initial treatment team seems to have considered treating his depression, anxiety, or nicotine disorders. While he did appear to abstain from both the opioids and alcohol for a few weeks or months after that initial discharge, he had not entered into any outpatient plan for recovery. He did not see himself as someone who could do a 12-step program, but he also didn't consider any of a number of other kinds of interventions. It also does not appear that progress was made in clarifying his work situation. Is he under investigation for stealing prescription opioids? Can he go back to work within his chosen profession? Should he go back to work in a field where pharmaceuticals are readily available? And, although it is crucial to take care of his core issues (suicidality, substance use, mood and anxiety), it is also important that someone get to know Dr. Kamin. What are his strengths? Who are his friends? Why did he have difficulty developing relationships prior to the onset of his opioid use disorder?

The dual diagnosis unit (i.e., the DDE) is essentially a psychiatric inpatient unit intertwined with evidence-based addiction treatment. The multidisciplinary treatment team offers traditional psychiatric treatment

**TABLE 13–1.** Applying the American Society of Addiction Medicine (ASAM) patient placement criteria to Dr. Kamin's case

| ASAM dimension | Assessment description | Dr. Kamin's assessment | Level of care |
|---|---|---|---|
| Dimension 1 | Acute intoxication and/or withdrawal potential | Although there are only mild signs or symptoms of withdrawal, recency of use and risks associated with alcohol withdrawal warrant careful monitoring and observation; additionally, dependence on two drug classes with serious withdrawal syndromes (alcohol, opioids) would likely necessitate a complicated detoxification regimen best rendered in an inpatient setting. | Level IV: inpatient, medically managed |
| Dimension 2 | Biomedical conditions and complications | Chronic back pain and difficulties in coping have resulted in an iatrogenic opioid dependence, the chronicity and severity of which significantly interfere with other aspects of treatment. | Level III: inpatient, medically monitored or Level IV: inpatient, medically managed |
| Dimension 3 | Emotional, behavioral, or cognitive conditions and complications | Complex and severe problems, including thoughts of self-harm, hopelessness, and an untreated mood disorder, constitute an imminent risk. | Level IV: inpatient, medically managed, dual diagnosis enhanced |

**TABLE 13–1.** Applying the American Society of Addiction Medicine (ASAM) patient placement criteria to Dr. Kamin's case *(continued)*

| ASAM dimension | Assessment description | Dr. Kamin's assessment | Level of care |
|---|---|---|---|
| Dimension 4 | Readiness to change | An attempt to seek treatment represents a transition to the "action" phase of change. However, relapse following recent residential treatment and a co-occurring illness suggest the need for more intensive engagement and motivational enhancement in a higher level of care. | Level III: inpatient, medically monitored or Level IV: inpatient, medically managed, dual diagnosis enhanced |
| Dimension 5 | Relapse, continued use or continued problem potential | Significant psychosocial stressors, including unemployment, lack of protective sober support networks, and untreated mental illness, indicate a high risk of continued use. | Level IV: inpatient, medically managed, dual diagnosis enhanced |
| Dimension 6 | Recovery/Living environment | Ease of access to drugs makes for a potentially toxic living/recovery environment. | Level III: inpatient/ residential or Level IV: inpatient, medically managed |

along with a variety of addiction treatments such as group therapy, motivational interviewing and motivational enhancement, specialized 12-step groups such as Double Trouble in Recovery meetings, and contingency management programs that allow patients to earn privileges during their stay. Physicians or nurse practitioners on the unit provide pharmacotherapy addressing both psychiatric and substance use disorders, with a particular interest in targeting cravings and helping to prevent relapse.

Recovery elements are often part of the unit structure. For example, the Serenity Prayer may be recited at the close of the daily community meeting, and wall murals may depict the Twelve Steps and Twelve Traditions. Music and art therapies can be especially effective for patients who are resistant to talk therapy and 12-step groups A final but key component of the DDE unit is specialized case management, which assists patients in coordinating discharge planning (Table 13–2).

In regard to Dr. Kamin, he will likely be offered an inpatient program that involves all of the modalities noted above.

**TABLE 13–2.   Components of a dual diagnosis inpatient unit**

| Modality | Discipline |
| --- | --- |
| Group therapy | All staff |
| Motivational interviewing/ Motivational enhancement therapy | All staff |
| Cognitive-behavioral therapy | Physicians, psychologists, social workers, counselors |
| 12-step groups | Nonpatient guests from the community |
| Contingency management | All staff |
| Music/Art therapy | Counselors, creative arts therapists, recreational therapists |
| Pharmacotherapy (for psychiatric and substance use disorders) | Physicians, nurse practitioners |
| Case management | Nurses, social workers |

## Psychotherapeutic and Psychosocial Interventions

### Group Therapy

Group therapy is a core treatment on many or most inpatient units, including a dual diagnosis unit. Psychoeducation and skills training groups are similar to those on general units, but DDE groups tend to focus on cravings and relapse prevention. As discussed further below, techniques such as motivational interviewing (MI) and cognitive-behavioral therapy (CBT) can also be woven into the groups.

### Motivational Interviewing and Motivational Enhancement Therapy

Patient motivation is a necessary component in the process of effecting change. Evidence indicates that MI can have a beneficial effect on SUDs, offering an efficient way to increase the frequency of healthy behaviors, decrease the frequency of unhealthy behaviors, and increase engagement in treatment (Lundahl et al. 2010).

Although evidence is limited, MI appears to work well on the inpatient unit. For example, one study found that a single session of MI in a drug detoxification setting led to increased patient self-efficacy and a greater likelihood that patients would transition to the preparation and action stages of recovery (Berman et al. 2010). In a recent randomized controlled trial, it was found that men with psychiatric disorders or dual diagnosis were at least 9.5 times more likely to show up to the first postdischarge appointment if they had received brief MI while hospitalized (Pantalon et al. 2014).

See Chapter 12, "Motivational Interviewing," for further discussion of MI.

### Cognitive-Behavioral Therapy

CBT has a long tradition of use in psychiatric treatment, and it can be a valuable tool in a dual diagnosis inpatient unit. In this setting, a CBT approach helps the patient to recognize and make plans to avoid high-risk situations, and to cope more effectively with urges and problems that arise during recovery (Carroll 2015). A "functional analysis" of drug use directs the patient to examine her or his use in meticulous detail—factors leading up to it, resulting consequences, and so forth. Skills training then provides the tools that the patient can use to put this knowledge to work. The following issues are often major focal points in a CBT approach: managing cravings, attending to early predictors of relapse, developing alternative coping skills, modifying overly guilty or unhealthy reactions to relapses, dismantling cognitive distortions about substance use (both positive and negative), and creating plans for lapses and relapses (Horsfall et al. 2009).

## 12-Step Groups

Traditional 12-step programs and mutual help organizations such as Alcoholics Anonymous (AA) have long been viewed as beneficial adjuncts to the comprehensive treatment of substance use disorders (Collins and Barth 1979). Increased attendance in 12-step groups has been associated with a higher proportion of abstinence, less severe distress, and fewer psychiatric symptoms (Moos et al. 1999). Their use and efficacy in the treatment of SUDs among the dually diagnosed, however, are less clearly established. Illness-related factors such as cognitive impairment, social anxiety, and paranoia may preclude dually diagnosed patients from effective participation in traditional AA meetings and lead to underutilization of mutual help services. Certain aspects of the AA philosophy may in fact be counterproductive to the recovery of some people with CODs. The use of confrontation as therapeutic strategy, for example, may be stress-provoking and increase the risk of relapse among vulnerable patients. Some people within the 12-step program may suggest the eschewal of all substances, including prescribed psychotropics. While the "anti-prescription" subgroup within 12-step has been diminishing for many years, this attitude can affect individuals with serious CODs and may lead to non-adherence and decompensation. Programs such as Double Trouble in Recovery, Dual Diagnosis Anonymous (Vogel et al. 1998) and Dual Recovery Anonymous (Hazelden Foundation 1993; Magura 2005; Substance Abuse and Mental Health Services Administration 2005) have emerged in recognition of these limitations of traditional 12-step programs for the dually diagnosed. Aiming to provide a more welcoming mutual health community for such patients, these programs have sought to adapt the mutual help recovery model of AA to the particular needs of the dually diagnosed.

Twelve-step programs are discussed in more detail in Chapter 11 ("Twelve-Step Programs").

## Contingency Management

Contingency management has much empirical support for being an effective strategy to help reinforce behaviors that promote drug abstinence. In the outpatient setting, reinforcement is achieved by offering rewards such as cash in the form of vouchers and prize draws shortly after confirmation of abstinence (e.g., by the finding of a negative urine drug screen at a clinic visit or a negative alcohol breath test). Studies have shown a high degree of efficacy compared with nonmonetary reinforcers for treatment of multiple drugs of abuse, including marijuana, alcohol, and tobacco, and in special populations such as marijuana-using adolescents and pregnant women who use tobacco (Galanter et al. 2015). Contingency management is applied in the inpatient setting using nonmonetary rewards to promote positive behavioral change by increasing independence. This strategy can be implemented through a "level system," for example, by which more access to certain recreational activities (e.g., going outside, having roof access, visiting a hospital shop) is allowed as a patient achieves higher levels.

## Music and Art Therapy

Music and art therapy have become common components of inpatient dual diagnosis units. While evidence is limited, music therapy on an inpatient psychiatric unit appears to improve mood, promote calm, and increase friendliness and to reduce both aggression and anxiety (Silverman and Rosenow 2013). In one study, even individuals with severe CODs were able to engage in music therapy (Ross et al. 2008); that same study (which took place on a dual diagnosis unit), found a link between greater attendance in music therapy sessions with a greater likelihood of attendance at the first aftercare appointment.

Group art therapy also suffers from a lack of empirical evidence, but anecdotal evidence suggests positive support from patients and staff alike for both music and art therapy.

## PHARMACOTHERAPY FOR PSYCHIATRIC AND SUBSTANCE USE DISORDERS

Dr. Kamin has multiple diagnoses, including a mood disorder (e.g., major depressive disorder) and a possible anxiety disorder. These diagnoses co-occur with alcohol, opioid, and tobacco use disorders. The inpatient service will likely be most acutely interested in assessing and managing safety, which would include the prevention of both suicide and serious alcohol withdrawal. Dr. Kamin lacks a known history of alcohol withdrawal but does admit to drinking 1 pint of alcohol per day. The inpatient protocol for such a patient varies significantly. In some hospitals, he would be observed and benzodiazepines would be initiated if significant withdrawal occurred. In other hospitals, benzodiazepines would be immediately initiated, with further doses as needed, and then tapered. In still others, a medication like clonidine would be started.

While acute alcohol withdrawal is being observed and managed, Dr. Kamin's clinicians will likely be considering a combined pharmacological approach to his CODs. Selective serotonin reuptake inhibitors (SSRIs) are the usual first-line treatment for depression in this population. Although perhaps slightly less effective than tricyclic antidepressants, SSRIs are better tolerated and accompanied by fewer adverse effects. While SSRIs can improve major depressions that are co-occurring with SUDs, the antidepressant appears to decrease the substance abuse only if the patient's mood improves first (Galanter et al. 2015). Rather than simply starting to take an antidepressant medication, Dr. Kamin should probably concurrently start treatment for alcohol use disorder. A combination of an SSRI and naltrexone has been found to produce improved alcohol abstinence, delay return to heavy drinking, and yield improvements in depressed mood among depressed alcoholics (Pettinati et al. 2010).

Tobacco is doubly problematic for Dr. Kamin. Not only does cigarette smoking lead to well-known medical complications, but continued use appears to increase the likelihood of an alcohol relapse. Tobacco use is acutely problematic on the inpatient unit because of the "no smoking" policy of hospitals, the frequency of co-occurring nicotine use disorder among people admitted with other CODs, and the drug's intense withdrawal effects. Inpatient hospitalizations can easily get derailed if newly admitted patients become preoccupied by the need for a cigarette, so it behooves inpatient clinicians to have a proactive plan to work with nicotine addiction (Ait-Daoud et al. 2006). Evidence is mixed in regard to pharmacological interventions for combined nicotine and alcohol use disorders. For example, nicotine replacement therapy (NRT) is a popular choice on inpatient units. Including nicotine gum and nicotine patches, NRT helps reduce craving in people who smoke cigarettes, but the effect appears to be diminished in those with a co-occurring alcohol use disorder (Karam-Hage et al. 2014).

In addition to its antidepressant effects, bupropion appears to help those who have recently stopped drinking to also stop smoking (Karam-Hage et al. 2014). Bupropion does not appear, however, to independently treat alcohol use disorder (Ait-Daoud et al. 2006) and has not been found to be more effective for smoking cessation in combination with NRT than NRT alone (Cahill et al. 2013).

Varenicline is a nicotinic receptor partial agonist that is also widely used by people trying to stop smoking. Evidence in the dual diagnosis population is limited, and there has been concern about varenicline worsening psychiatric symptoms and suicidality. A recent meta-analysis, however, focusing on smokers with serious mental illness showed varenicline to be effective and tolerable for smoking cessation (Roberts et al. 2016).

Pharmacotherapy for Dr. Kamin's opioid use disorder appears to be crucial. Medication-assisted treatment (MAT) would likely be the most effective medication treatment for Dr. Kamin's opioid use disorder. MAT includes the opioid agonist maintenance therapies methadone and buprenorphine, and the opioid antagonist therapy naltrexone (available orally or by depot injection). For opioid use disorders in general, MAT is the gold standard (Sees et al. 2000; Zerbo and Aggarwal 2016). This has been established by several studies and a wealth of clinical data, which demonstrate clearly that nonpharmacological interventions used alone are not as effective as MAT (Mattick et al. 2009). Dr. Kamin is at particular risk. Like many people with opioid use disorder, Dr. Kamin relapsed after his previous hospitalization. Overdose deaths are a major public health issue in the United States, with a quadrupling of deaths between 1999 and 2014. Prescription sales of opioids have also quadrupled during that time frame, and, as we see with Dr. Kamin, a typical pattern of opioid use has shifted from urban minorities to suburban whites. And, as with Dr. Kamin., it is not uncommon for people to shift their use from prescribed opioids to heroin because heroin is cheaper (Cicero et al. 2014).

## SPECIALIZED CASE MANAGEMENT

Major obstacles to successful treatment are a disruptive home and community environment and the lack of coordinated care. Specialized case management helps to provide coordinated services to at-risk patient populations (Center for Behavioral Health Statistics and Quality 2015). Case managers have typically been trained as social workers or nurses, though such individuals can have a variety of backgrounds. Administrative advocates and psychological sources of support, case managers assist with such issues as housing, employment, and finances. On an inpatient unit, their early participation is crucial. Acquisition of social services can take days or weeks, for example, and so discharge can be delayed. Delays are costly to the hospital, but they can also impede the patient's transfer to a rehab facility and/or increase the likelihood of a postdischarge relapse, which can, in turn, lead to a revolving door of hospital admissions. In other words, robust case management services are not only clinically useful but also a cost-effective part of the treatment team.

## INCORPORATING DUAL DIAGNOSIS ELEMENTS INTO THE GENERAL PSYCHIATRIC UNIT

Although dual diagnosis units exist around the country, the large majority of people with CODs who need an acute psychiatric admission are admitted to general psychiatric units. General psychiatric units can provide many of the same services as a dedicated unit, which is important since, nationwide, half of those admitted to a psychiatric unit also have an SUD. Needs vary between hospital populations, but it appears that a more holistic and integrated approach can reduce some of the barriers to successful treatment (Center for Mental Health Services 2009). A free multimedia kit entitled "Integrated Treatment for Co-Occurring Disorders (Evidence-Based Practices)" (Center for Mental Health Services 2009) can help guide clinicians who would like to integrate their usual inpatient practices with the treatment of SUDs.

# Conclusion

Inpatient treatment has a special place within the spectrum of substance abuse treatment; although it accounts for a small percentage of overall treatment admissions, it is the most intensive setting and involves treating the most medically and psychiatrically complicated patients. In this chapter, we focused on the inpatient dual diagnosis unit found in a hospital setting, which is an even more specialized type of inpatient treatment that has received little attention in the literature. Although there is a much smaller number of these units as compared with general psychiatric units, the components can be exported to general units for more specialized treatment of the dual diagnosis population. Given that a large number of psychiatric inpatients are actually dual diagnosis patients, it is critical that these components be incorporated in order to provide the most effective treatment possible and to enhance recovery rates upon discharge.

## KEY POINTS

- Almost half of all admissions for substance abuse treatment are to a non-ambulatory environment, and almost half of those patients admitted for treatment to all substance abuse settings had a co-occurring mental health diagnosis.

- The ASAM Patient Placement Criteria provide a structured method to assess patients for the appropriate level of care, involving six dimensions of assessment and five broad levels of care.

- While there are a variety of specialized components utilized on a "gold standard" dual diagnosis inpatient unit, many of these can be incorporated into a general psychiatric unit for use with patients with co-occurring disorders.

# Questions

1. Which of the following best describes a "gold standard" dual diagnosis inpatient unit?

    A. An inpatient detoxification unit with direct linkage to an inpatient psychiatry unit.
    B. An inpatient unit staffed by internists and psychiatrists in order to provide complete medical and psychiatric care.
    C. An inpatient unit employing motivation enhancement therapy, relapse prevention, contingency management, and 12-step group work.
    D. An inpatient unit with a focus on transitioning patients to long-term residential treatment upon discharge.

2. Based on the proposed taxonomy of addiction treatment programs discussed in this chapter and the ASAM patient placement criteria, an acutely suicidal patient at risk of alcohol withdrawal should be matched to which of the following treatment settings:

    A. Level III, Inpatient, medically monitored, Dual diagnosis enhanced.
    B. Level III, Residential, Addiction only services.
    C. Level IV, Inpatient medically managed, Dual diagnosis enhanced.
    D. Level III, Residential, Dual diagnosis capable.

3. Which of the following factors may limit the efficacy of traditional 12-step programs as recovery resource for the dually diagnosed and lead to underutilization of mutual help services?

    A. Confrontation as a therapeutic strategy.
    B. Illness-related factors such as cognitive impairment and paranoia.
    C. An "anti-prescription" bias.
    D. All of the above.

4. Which of the following forms of treatment discussed in this chapter have been found to increase the likelihood of showing up to the first postdischarge appointment?

   A. Cognitive-behavioral therapy.
   B. Motivational interviewing.
   C. Art therapy.
   D. Psychodynamic psychotherapy.

# References

Ait-Daoud N, Lynch WJ, Penberthy JK, et al: Treating smoking dependence in depressed alcoholics. Alcohol Res Health 29(3):213–220, 2006 17373412

Berman AH, Forsberg L, Durbeej N, et al: Single-session motivational interviewing for drug detoxification inpatients: effects on self-efficacy, stages of change and substance use. Subst Use Misuse 45(3):384–402, 2010 DOI: 10.3109/10826080903452488 20141454

Brunette MF, Mueser KT, Drake RE: A review of research on residential programs for people with severe mental illness and co-occurring substance use disorders. Drug Alcohol Rev 23(4):471–481, 2004 15763752

Cahill K, Stevens S, Perera R, Lancaster T: Pharmacological interventions for smoking cessation: an overview and network meta-analysis. Cochrane Database Syst Rev (5):CD009329, 2013 23728690

Carroll KM: Cognitive-behavioral therapies, in The American Psychiatric Publishing Textbook of Substance Abuse Treatment, 5th Edition. Edited by Galanter M, Kleber HD, Brady KT. Washington, DC, American Psychiatric Publishing, 2015, pp 385–395

Center for Behavioral Health Statistics and Quality: Treatment Episode Data Set (TEDS): 2003–2013. National Admissions to Substance Abuse Treatment Services. BHSIS Series S-75 (HHS Publ No SMA-15–4934). Rockville, MD, Substance Abuse and Mental Health Services Administration, 2015

Center for Mental Health Services: Integrated Treatment for Co-Occurring Disorders: The Evidence (DHHS Publ No SMA-08-4366). Rockville, MD, Substance Abuse and Mental Health Services Administration, U.S. Department of Health and Human Services, 2009. Available at: https://store.samhsa.gov/shin/content/SMA08-4367/TheEvidence-ITC.pdf. Accessed March 2, 2017.

Cicero TJ, Ellis MS, Surratt HL, et al: The changing face of heroin use in the United States: a retrospective analysis of the past 50 years. JAMA Psychiatry 71(7):821–826, 2014 24871348

Collins GB, Barth J: Using the resources of AA in treating alcoholics in a general hospital. Hosp Community Psychiatry 30(7):480–482, 1979 447233

Dickey B, Azeni H: Persons with dual diagnoses of substance abuse and major mental illness: their excess costs of psychiatric care. Am J Public Health 86(7):973–977, 1996 8669521

Galanter M, Kleber HD, Brady KT (eds): The American Psychiatric Publishing Textbook of Substance Abuse Treatment, 5th Edition. Washington, DC, American Psychiatric Publishing, 2015

Haywood TW, Kravitz HM, Grossman LS, et al: Predicting the "revolving door" phenomenon among patients with schizophrenic, schizoaffective, and affective disorders. Am J Psychiatry 152(6):856–861, 1995 7755114

Hazelden Foundation: The Dual Diagnosis Recovery Book. Center City, MN, Hazelden Foundation, 1993

Horsfall J, Cleary M, Hunt GE, et al: Psychosocial treatments for people with co-occurring severe mental illnesses and substance use disorders (dual diagnosis): a review of empirical evidence. Harv Rev Psychiatry 17(1):24–34, 2009 19205964

Karam-Hage M, Robinson JD, Lodhi A, et al: Bupropion-SR for smoking reduction and cessation in alcohol-dependent outpatients: a naturalistic, open-label study. Curr Clin Pharmacol 9(2):123–129, 2014 24218993

Lundahl B, Kunz C, Brownell C, et al: A meta-analysis of motivational interviewing: twenty-five years of empirical studies. Res Soc Work Pract 20(2):137–160, 2010

Magura S: Effectiveness of dual focus mutual aid for co-occurring substance use and mental health disorders: a review and synthesis of the "Double Trouble" in Recovery evaluation. Subst Use Misuse 43(12–13):1904–1926, 2008 2923916

Mattick RP, Breen C, Kimber J, et al: Methadone maintenance therapy versus no opioid replacement therapy for opioid dependence. Cochrane Database Syst Rev (3):CD002209, 2009 19588333

Mee-Lee D, Shulman GD, Fishman M (eds): ASAM Patient Placement Criteria for the Treatment of Substance-Related Disorders, 2nd Edition, Revised (ASAM PPC-2R). Chevy Chase, MD, American Society of Addiction Medicine, 2001

Moos RH, Finney JW, Ouimette PC, et al: A comparative evaluation of substance abuse treatment: I. Treatment orientation, amount of care, and 1-year outcomes. Alcohol Clin Exp Res 23(3):529–536, 1999 10195829

Moos RH, Finney JW, Moos BS: Inpatient substance abuse care and the outcome of subsequent community residential and outpatient care. Addiction 95(6):833–846, 2000 10946434

Oh Min M, Biegel D, Johnsen J: Predictors of psychiatric hospitalization for adults with co-occurring substance and mental disorders as compared to adults with mental illness only. Psychiatric Rehabilitation Journal 29(2):114–121, 2005

Pantalon MV, Murphy MK, Barry DT, et al: Predictors and moderators of aftercare appointment-keeping following brief motivational interviewing among patients with psychiatric disorders or dual diagnosis. J Dual Diagn 10(1):44–51, 2014 25392061

Pettinati H, Oslin D, Kampman K, et al: A double-blind, placebo-controlled trial combining sertraline and naltrexone for treating co-occurring depression and alcohol dependence. Am J Psychiatry 167(6):668–675, 2010 20231324

Ridgely MS, Goldman HH, Willenbring M: Barriers to the care of persons with dual diagnoses: organizational and financing issues. Schizophr Bull 16(1):123–132, 1990 2185535

Roberts E, Evins AE, McNeill A, et al: Efficacy and tolerability of pharmacotherapy for smoking cessation in adults with serious mental illness: a systematic review and network meta-analysis. Addiction 111(4):599–612, 2016 26594837

Ross S, Cidambi I, Dermatis H, et al: Music therapy: a novel motivational approach for dually diagnosed patients. J Addict Dis 27(1):41–53, 2008 18551887

Sees KL, Delucchi KL, Masson C, et al: Methadone maintenance vs 180-day psychosocially enriched detoxification for treatment of opioid dependence: a randomized controlled trial. JAMA 283(10):1303–1310, 2000 10714729

Sharon E, Krebs C, Turner W, et al: Predictive validity of the ASAM Patient Placement Criteria for hospital utilization. J Addict Dis 22(Suppl 1):79–93, 2003 15991591

Silverman M, Rosenow S: Immediate quantitative effects of recreational music therapy on mood and perceived helpfulness in acute psychiatric inpatients: an exploratory investigation. Arts Psychother 40(3):269–274, 2013

Stallvik M, Gastfriend DR: Predictive and convergent validity of the ASAM Criteria in Norway. Addict Res Theory 22(6):515–523, 2014

Substance Abuse and Mental Health Services Administration: Substance Abuse Treatment for Persons With Co-Occurring Disorders. Treatment Improvement Protocol (TIP) Series, No. 42. (HHS Publ No SMA-33992). Rockville, MD, Substance Abuse and Mental Health Services Administration, 2005

Vogel HS, Knight E, Laudet AB, et al: Double Trouble in Recovery: self-help for the dually diagnosed. Psychiatr Rehabil J 21(4):356–364, 1998 17710222

Zerbo E, Aggarwal R: Opioids, in Pocket Guide to Addiction Assessment and Treatment. Edited by Levounis P, Zerbo E, Aggarwal R. Arlington, VA, American Psychiatric Association Publishing, 2016, pp 171–200

# 14

# PHARMACOLOGICAL INTERVENTIONS

## Jonathan D. Avery, M.D.

This chapter highlights important pharmacological treatments for patients with co-occurring disorders (CODs) with a focus on medications for substance use disorders (SUDs). While a range of clinicians feel comfortable offering medications to patients to treat anxiety disorders, major depressive disorder, and other psychiatric disorders, medical professionals often feel they have little in the way of medications to treat individuals' SUDs. As a result, individuals with CODs often have their mental illness alone treated with medications. Historically, 12-step groups and other psychosocial interventions have dominated the addiction treatment landscape, and these treatment modalities have, at times, discouraged medications for SUDs as well.

There are several safe, effective, and easy-to-administer medications, however, that may improve outcomes for individuals with SUDs, with and without CODs. Table 14–1 provides a summary of some of these medications. Most can be administered to individuals with a range of psychiatric diagnoses and have minimal interactions with psychotropic medications. As a result, these medications for SUDs can be easily incorporated into the interventions that are offered to patients with CODs.

The following case will highlight some of the common opportunities physicians will encounter to prescribe medications for patients' CODs.

---

## Clinical Case

Dr. Allen is a 39-year-old psychiatrist with a history of referring individuals with SUDs to 12-step programs or other providers.

Dr. Allen's first patient of the day, Elena, surprises him by reporting that she would like a medication to help her curb her cravings for alcohol and weekend binges. Dr. Allen had been treating Elena's major depressive disorder and social anxiety disorder with citalopram and weekly therapy for many years. At times, they would discuss her history of heavy alcohol use during college and her regrets about this time, but she had not brought it up recently. Because of her social anxiety and busy work schedule, she is not interested in groups or additional treatment modalities.

Dr. Allen's second patient of the day, Ernesto, reports he is finally ready to quit cigarettes. He has been diagnosed with bipolar I disorder and has been stable while taking lithium and olanzapine for several years. Ernesto says he has tried to quit on his own for many months by using a nicotine patch and gum and even tried hypnosis, but now he is ready "to get serious" about it. He saw a commercial for varenicline and would like to start it right away.

Dr. Allen's third patient of the day is a new evaluation. Ashley is a 26-year-old woman with a history of opioid use disorder and schizophrenia, and she is hoping to find an antipsychotic medication that does not interact with methadone. She reports that she has started to work again and regained a lot of her function since enrolling in a methadone clinic several months ago, but reports that paranoia and auditory hallucinations are impairing her ability to engage appropriately with people at work and in her life.

**TABLE 14–1. Medications for substance use disorders (with average doses)**

| Tobacco use disorder | Alcohol use disorder | Opioid use disorder |
|---|---|---|
| Varenicline (Chantix) 1 mg po BID | Naltrexone (ReVia) 50 mg po QD | Buprenorphine[a] (Suboxone) 8–16 mg SL QD |
| Bupropion (Wellbutrin, Zyban) 150 mg po BID | (Vivitrol) 380 mg IM Qmonth | Methadone (Dolophine, Methadose) 60–120 mg po QD |
| Nicotine replacement therapies | Acamprosate (Campral) 666 mg po TID | Naltrexone (ReVia) 50 mg po QD |
| | Disulfiram (Antabuse) 125–500 mg po QD | (Vivitrol) 380 mg IM Qmonth |
| | Topiramate (Topamax) 75–150 mg po BID | |
| | Gabapentin (Neurontin) 600–1,200 mg po daily | |

*Note.*   BID=twice a day; IM=intramuscularly; Q=every; QD=once a day; po=by mouth; TID=three times a day; SL=sublingually.
[a]Usually combined with naloxone, and available in several forms and preparations (film, tablet, implants).

# Discussion

Dr. Allen is treating three patients with rather common presentations. After all, alcohol and tobacco use disorders are very prevalent among individuals with mental illness. Clinicians often worry about treating individuals with methadone or buprenorphine because of drug-drug interactions and concerns about how to best integrate substance use treatments like a methadone program. We will discuss these issues further in the section "Treatment" below.

Dr. Allen is also like many other physicians who do not routinely offer medications for SUDs but rather focus on treating the co-occurring psychiatric disorders. In one study in the U.S. Veterans Affairs healthcare system, for example, only 7%–11% of patients received medications for their alcohol use disorder, while 69%–82% received medications for the co-occurring psychiatric disorder (Rubinsky et al. 2015). The reasons behind this reluctance to prescribe medications for SUDs are likely many and include lack of knowledge about such medications, rejection of the disease model of addiction, and stigmatizing attitudes toward individuals with SUDs (Avery et al. 2017).

With the current opioid epidemic and high number of fatal overdoses from opioids, the reluctance to prescribe medications for opioid use disorder is especially problematic. Starting opioid agonist therapy after an overdose, for example, has been associated with a 50% reduction in subsequent death, yet less than 5% of those who survive an overdose receive pharmacotherapy (Massachusetts Department of Public Health 2016). Further, studies have shown that opioid agonist therapy is effective even without additional psychosocial interventions (Wakeman 2017).

The idea of incorporating medications into the treatment of SUDs is fairly recent, though, because psychosocial interventions have predominated for many years. Twelve-step programs for recovery, such as Alcoholics Anonymous (AA) and Narcotics Anonymous (NA), have often been considered first-line treatments (see Chapter 11, "Twelve-Step Programs"). These programs are mutual help groups that are not run by physicians or therapists, and as a result, medications for the treatment of substance use disorders are often not addressed. In fact, although not an official position of AA, at times members have claimed that medications are not to be used to support sobriety (Mendola and Gibson 2016). Nonmedication stances can be taken by practitioners of other psychosocial treatments as well, including those practicing motivational interviewing and cognitive-behavioral therapy.

The challenge for clinicians like Dr. Allen is that it is not clear as of yet which patients will benefit most from medications alone, psychosocial treatments alone, or a combination of treatment modalities (Mendola and Gibson 2016). There is enough evidence, however, to strongly recommend using medications for at least tobacco, alcohol, and opioid use disorders.

# Treatment

The focus below is on the treatment of tobacco use disorder, alcohol use disorder, and opioid use disorder in individuals with co-occurring psychiatric disorders. There is unfortunately limited evidence for medications for other SUDs as of yet. It is important to note that in the following discussion the assumption is that the co-occurring psychiatric disorder is also being treated with the appropriate medications and psychosocial treatments. As discussed above, the treatment of the psychiatric disorder is often what comes first, and the treatment of these co-occurring SUDs is what is ignored or deferred.

## TOBACCO USE DISORDER

Ernesto in the above case has both a serious mental illness and a tobacco use disorder, which is a very common clinical presentation. While the treatment of such individuals often focuses first on adequately treating the mental illness, the medical complications from tobacco use can just as easily lead to decreased quality of life, morbidity, and mortality.

Treatment of tobacco use disorder ideally combines behavioral interventions and pharmacological interventions. The first-line pharmacological interventions include nicotine replacement therapy (NRT), varenicline, and bupropion. These medications, however, have a long history of not being prescribed to individuals with psychiatric disorders because of concern that they may make psychiatric symptoms worse.

The data highlight that the neuropsychiatric adverse events from these medications are few and should be prescribed to individuals with CODs. A large, recent study of more than 4,000 subjects with psychiatric disorders and 4,000 without, for example, did not show a significant increase in neuropsychiatric adverse events attributable to varenicline or bupropion relative to nicotine patch or placebo and demonstrated the efficacy of these medications (Anthenelli et al. 2016). Bupropion, of course, has the added benefit of potentially treating depressive symptoms as well.

It is important to keep in mind though that the byproducts of tobacco smoking induce cytochrome P450 (CYP) 1A2, and thus stopping smoking may lead to increases in the levels of antipsychotics such as clozapine, olanzapine, and haloperidol.

Dr. Allen should feel comfortable, as a result, prescribing varenicline to Ernesto. Dr. Allen will have to monitor for side effects of olanzapine as Ernesto stops smoking, though, and may have to lower the dose.

## ALCOHOL USE DISORDER

Elena is another example of someone who would benefit from medications for all of her diagnoses. Her social situation and anxiety symptoms are such that she does not want to participate in 12-step programs or other psychosocial treatments. She has a long-standing relationship with Dr. Allen and is interested in additional medications to help her curb her cravings and alcohol use.

Table 14–1 lists medications that may be helpful for individuals with alcohol use disorder, and Table 14–2 details the few contraindications to these medications. Disulfiram has been integrated into substance use treatments for many years and seems to work best when individuals are motivated to maintain abstinence or are supervised when they take it to ensure compliance. Oral naltrexone and long-acting injectable naltrexone have become increasingly utilized and help with craving, abstinence, and moderation. Acamprosate has the advantage of being metabolized by the kidney, although the data for its use are not as strong as for naltrexone. The use of these medications in individuals with particular mental illnesses is discussed throughout this book, and they are easily combined with psychotropic medications without concern for interactions or neuropsychiatric side effects (Seneviratne and Johnson 2015).

The use of gabapentin and topiramate for alcohol use disorder is especially promising for individuals with CODs because these medications also have evidence for treating mental illnesses. Both are thought to potentially help with mood and anxiety, although certainly the level of evidence is not the same as that for antidepressants or more classic mood stabilizers, and topiramate may be helpful for individuals with borderline personality disorder as well (Stoffers et al. 2010).

Dr. Allen could easily add naltrexone to Elena's medications to target her cravings and bingeing behaviors. If she were unable to moderate her use and wanted to stop drinking altogether, Dr. Allen could then add disulfiram, potentially bringing in Elena's significant other to the treatment to set up daily supervised administration of the medication.

**TABLE 14–2.** Contraindications to medications for alcohol use disorder[a]

| Medication | Contraindications |
|---|---|
| Naltrexone | Opioid use, acute hepatitis, severe liver disease |
| Acamprosate | Severe renal impairment |
| Disulfiram | Alcohol, metronidazole, severe cardiac disease |
| Topiramate | None |
| Gabapentin | None |

[a]These agents are generally avoided in pregnancy, although data are limited. Topiramate is category D (positive evidence of risk).

## Opioid Use Disorder

Ashley has both a mental illness and an opioid use disorder and would benefit from medications for both. As discussed earlier, opioid use disorders are unique in that evidence for medication-assisted treatment is so strong and potentially life-saving (Wakeman 2017).

Methadone, buprenorphine, or naltrexone—especially long-acting, injectable naltrexone—is the standard of treatment, with the evidence being strongest for methadone and buprenorphine. As discussed earlier, naltrexone has few side effects and interactions with other medications. There are several things to keep in mind with methadone and buprenorphine.

As in the case of Ashley, methadone is prescribed as part of an opioid treatment program. It is a full opioid agonist. As with any other opioid, one has to be careful with medications that cause respiratory depression (such as benzodiazepines). Methadone is also metabolized by enzymes in the CYP system (particularly CYP3A4) and interacts with many medications (Shinderman et al. 2003). Table 14–3 describes some of the effects of psychotropic medications on methadone levels; similarly, methadone can alter the levels of other medications. Methadone also prolongs the corrected QT interval. Ideally, a clinician treating an individual taking methadone will be in close contact with that person's treatment team at the methadone clinic so that each party is aware of changes to medications and the potential impact on the individual.

Buprenorphine is a partial opioid agonist that is also metabolized by the CYP3A4 system. It does not appear to prolong the corrected QT in-

**TABLE 14–3.  Selected effects of psychotropic medications on methadone levels**

| Reduce methadone levels | Phenobarbital, carbamazepine |
| Increase methadone levels | Sertraline, amitriptyline, paroxetine, fluvoxamine, diazepam, alprazolam |

terval to the same degree as methadone. It can be administered alone or in combination with the opioid antagonist naloxone, which is active if used intravenously and in theory protects against such abuse. Buprenorphine can be administered in a clinician's office, and a range of medical professionals are completing the training course and registration in order to prescribe it to their patients. The induction and maintenance of buprenorphine are rather straight-forward; one sample induction schedule is shown in Table 14–4. As with methadone, clinicians have to be mindful of drug-drug interactions and the risk for respiratory depression and misuse. Again, though, the risks of not treating (including death) are much greater that the risk and side effects of treating (Avery 2011; Wakeman 2017).

Dr. Allen may elect for Ashley to start taking aripiprazole, as it has fewer drug-drug interactions with methadone and less corrected QT interval prolongation than other antipsychotic medications. He should also plan on staying in contact with her methadone program so that they can keep each other informed of dose changes along the way.

# Conclusion

It is important to offer individuals with CODs treatment options for all their conditions. While medication options to treat psychiatric disorders are in many cases employed, medications are often not prescribed to treat individuals' SUDs. When medications are used for all disorders, the clinician must keep in mind interactions between the different medications.

## KEY POINTS

- Individuals with co-occurring disorders often have their mental illness alone treated with medications.

**TABLE 14–4.** Sample buprenorphine induction—first 2 days

| Day 1 | | Day 2 | | Day 3 |
|---|---|---|---|---|
| First dose | Next dose | First dose | Next dose | Day 3 |
| 2–4 mg when in at least moderate opioid withdrawal | Redose in 1–3 hours for continued withdrawal symptoms up to a total of 12 mg | Give Day 1 total dosage | For continued withdrawal later in day, give additional 2–4 mg | Give Day 2 total dosage |

- There are effective medications for tobacco, alcohol, and opioid use disorders.
- Psychotropic medications metabolized by the cytochrome P450 system may impact levels of methadone and buprenorphine.

# Questions

1. Approximately what percentage of individuals with substance use disorders (SUDs) receive pharmacological treatment for their SUD?

    A. 10%.
    B. 25%.
    C. 50%.
    D. 75%.

2. Which of the following medications may treat both an individual's personality disorder and his or her SUD?

    A. Gabapentin.
    B. Topiramate.
    C. Disulfiram.
    D. Naltrexone.

3. Which of the following is a contraindication to starting naltrexone?

    A. Current depressive episode.
    B. Renal impairment.
    C. Severe liver failure.
    D. Current treatment with escitalopram.

# References

Anthenelli RM, Benowitz NL, West R, et al: Neuropsychiatric safety and efficacy of varenicline, bupropion, and nicotine patch in smokers with and without psychiatric disorders (EAGLES): a double-blind, randomised, placebo-controlled clinical trial. Lancet 387(10037):2507–2520, 2016 27116918

Avery JD: A resident's guide to buprenorphine. American Journal of Psychiatry Residents' Journal 6(9):3–5, 2011

Avery J, Han BH, Zerbo E, et al: Changes in psychiatry residents' attitudes towards individuals with substance use disorders over the course of residency training. Am J Addict 26(1):75–79, 2017 27749984

Massachusetts Department of Public Health: An assessment of opioid-related deaths in Massachusetts, September 15, 2016. Available at: http://www.mass.gov/eohhs/docs/dph/stop-addiction/chapter-55-opioid-overdose-study-data-brief-9–15–2016.pdf. Accessed February 7, 2017.

Mendola A, Gibson RL: Addiction, 12-step programs, and evidentiary standards for ethically and clinically sound treatment recommendations: what should clinicians do? AMA J Ethics 18(6):646–655, 2016 27322999

Rubinsky AD, Chen C, Batki SL, et al: Comparative utilization of pharmacotherapy for alcohol use disorder and other psychiatric disorders among U.S. Veterans Health Administration patients with dual diagnoses. J Psychiatr Res 69:150–157, 2015 26343607

Seneviratne C, Johnson BA: Advances in medications and tailoring treatment for alcohol use disorder. Alcohol Res 37(1):15–28, 2015 26259086

Shinderman M, Maxwell S, Brawand-Amey M, et al: Cytochrome P4503A4 metabolic activity, methadone blood concentrations, and methadone doses. Drug Alcohol Depend 69(2):205–211, 2003 12609702

Stoffers J, Völlm BA, Rücker G, et al: Pharmacological interventions for borderline personality disorder. Cochrane Database Syst Rev (6):CD005653, 2010 20556762

Wakeman SE: Medications for addiction treatment: changing the language to improve care. J Addict Med 11(1):1–2, 2017 27898497

# PART 4

## SPECIAL POPULATIONS

# 15

# ADOLESCENCE

## Shannon G. Caspersen, M.D., M.Phil.

The evaluation and treatment of adolescent substance use disorders (SUDs) and co-occurring mental illness is different from that of adults in a variety of ways. First, the treatment of the adolescent inevitably involves the family. Regardless of whether they are still legal minors, adolescents are generally still dependent financially, emotionally, and logistically on their parents. Therefore, the patient cannot be treated in a vacuum; instead, the whole family must be engaged for the treatment to be successful.

A second issue revolves around the fact that adolescents are more impulsive than adults and less able to plan and make executive decisions. Much of the difference can be linked to the maturation of the nervous system (Tau and Peterson 2010). Heavily implicated in complex decision making, impulse control, and emotional regulation, the prefrontal cortex matures relatively late. The earlier-maturing nucleus accumbens (ventral striatum) is a target of mesolimbic dopamine projections and therefore plays a central role in reward and addiction; it is more active than the prefrontal cortex during adolescence, effectively overwhelming it (Casey and Jones 2010). Moreover, the amygdala's fear response is less active during adolescence than it is during childhood and adulthood, so that risk-avoidance is reduced during the adolescent period compared with childhood and adulthood (Ernst 2014). The net result of the three different developmental trajectories of the prefrontal cortex and amygdala on the one hand and the ventral striatum on the other is that the impulsivity of the reward system is more powerful than the fear response of the amygdala and the control response of the prefrontal cortex. Risk, reward, and cognitive control are imbalanced.

A third difference between adolescents and adults relates to confidentiality laws. Just as it is with adult patients, psychotherapy can be negatively affected when the patient does not trust that confidentiality will be maintained. In both adults and minors, confidential information can be revealed under court order, with the patient's permission, and/or when there appears to be a danger to self or others. In addition, both groups lose the right to confidentiality when they agree in advance to a forensics exam. These rules hold for the adolescent, but there are times when the courts and parents may need to hear a "metabolized" version of events, over the patient's objection, even when the patient's life is not at risk, for treatment planning and implementation purposes. The laws vary state by state, and there is a certain amount of ambiguity that can relate to the minor's age and level of independence, but the clinician will need to be aware of local rules before guaranteeing absolute privacy to a wary adolescent.

The following case illustrates some of these age-specific considerations in the assessment and treatment of adolescents with co-occurring disorders (CODs).

---

## Clinical Case

Dara is a 17-year-old eleventh-grade girl who is referred from her pediatrician to a child psychiatrist because her grades have dropped and she has been unable to efficiently finish her homework. Her parents want her to be assessed for attention-deficit/hyperactivity disorder (ADHD) and the potential need for stimulant medication and additional time on school tests and the SAT.

Dara's parents describe her as a popular, "A" student who has been struggling academically for about a year. They also note that she seems to care less about her grades than she has in the past, which they attribute to her joining a less ambitious peer group. Dara herself reports significant anxiety related to academic stress and pressure from her parents to get into a good college, as her parents and older brother attended the same elite college. She adds that she wants to be an actress, but her parents expect her to be "gung ho for law school." She does admit that she used to like school but now finds her school-work too difficult. After being reminded of the confidentiality of the sessions, Dara admits that the main way she gets relief from stress is to smoke cannabis with friends. She believes that "weed" not only relieves her anxiety but also helps her sleep, so she uses it before going to bed, using a vaporizer pen so that her parents do not smell it. She finds herself daydreaming about "party-ing" when she should be concentrating on class. When asked about her ability to complete homework, she admits to feeling overwhelmed. She has difficulty organizing essays and keeping track of homework assignments. She adds that this feeling of disorganization makes her more anxious and therefore more intent on using cannabis in order to relax.

Dara describes her cannabis use as "part of the solution, not part of the problem." She started using cannabis with friends at age 13 and for the past few years has been "doing fine." She identifies her problem as related not to cannabis but instead to her parents' overly high expectations. To deal with this stress during the school day, she typically "vapes" at lunchtime, after school with friends, and again before going to bed to help her sleep. On the weekends, she vapes several times in the after-noon and evening while hanging out with her friends and her boyfriend, all of whom use cannabis. She describes the canna-bis as being "great for sleep" but acknowledges that she has been unable to get to school on time and that she has been suspended from the drama club for missing Saturday morning rehearsals.

Dara denies all symptoms of depression, mania, psycho-sis, eating disorder, suicidal thoughts, and self-injury.

In addition to cannabis use, Dara reports smoking five to-bacco cigarettes per day for 2–3 years. Nicotine helps her con-centrate, she says, and also covers up the smell of cannabis. She reports drinking about three beers per weekend at par-ties, starting at age 12, but has never vomited or blacked out from alcohol. She has tried cocaine once and ecstasy twice, but those drugs aren't readily available through her friends. She denies recreational use of any prescription medications or other illicit drugs.

With regard to risk behaviors that have occurred while intoxicated, Dara insists that she has never driven a car while under the influence of alcohol or other drugs, but she does report jumping between subway cars on a dare once while under the influence of cannabis. She also admits to having accidentally started a fire in her bedroom by leaving a "blunt" burning on her bed. She has had unprotected intercourse with her boyfriend numerous times while under the influence of cannabis, but she has always used protection when not intoxicated.

Dara states that her parents would "flip out" if they learned how much she smokes, but that she herself thinks it is "no big deal" because marijuana is a natural plant that everyone uses. She says that she mainly smokes because it feels good and to deal with the stress that her parents put her under via the pressure they place on her to perform.

# Discussion

While Dara denies having difficulties, her marijuana use still meets DSM-5 criteria for a SUD. She spends a lot of time acquiring, using, and recovering from the substance; she craves the substance; she is unable to manage her responsibilities at home and school; she has given up her primary extracurricular activity (drama) in favor of getting high; and she has recurrently put herself into danger while intoxicated.

The history of symptom onset is particularly important in clarifying the ADHD diagnosis. It appears that Dara's ability to focus, organize, and efficiently finish assignments was fine until age 16 and then markedly declined. ADHD is typically recognized earlier, and even if the diagnosis is not made until later, problems can generally be recognized in retrospect. For this reason, DSM-5 suggests that attentional symptoms in ADHD should be recognized prior to age 12, a criterion that Dara's case does not meet. The temporal association between her clinical symptoms and her marijuana use makes ADHD even more unlikely.

An ADHD diagnosis is made more complicated by the potential for secondary gain. Even well-meaning patients and parents can try to push for an ADHD diagnosis when they perceive the possibility of additional time on standardized tests and the availability of performance-enhancing stimulants. As part of a careful and tactful clinical interview, questionnaires such as the Vanderbilt Assessment Scales (Wolraich et al. 1998) can help distinguish between clinically significant ADHD and subclinical attentional difficulties. To elucidate whether the inattention the patient is experiencing is primary or secondary to cannabis use, the clinician could use these scales at baseline and then repeat them after the patient has achieved a period of abstinence.

In regard to Dara's school difficulties, it appears clear that heavy substance use during adolescence can have a marked effect on learning, attention, retention, and psychomotor processing speed (Rosner 2013). These effects occur not just during intoxication (Rosner 2013). Even after a month of abstinence from cannabis, adolescent users have still been found to have impaired memory, working memory, planning, and sequencing abilities (Jacobus et al. 2009; Medina et al. 2007). Dara complains that she has difficulty focusing, planning, organizing, and finishing assignments. These difficulties can all be attributed to marijuana use more easily than to a late onset of ADHD.

While ADHD appears unlikely in Dara, it is possible that she has a diagnosis on the anxiety spectrum. She describes increasing amounts of anxiety during high school, and like other adolescents, she seems to view her cannabis use as a way to relax (Buckner and Schmidt 2008). Cannabis use can diminish anxiety acutely, but it can also worsen anxiety, particularly in the withdrawal state that can be felt within a day of not smoking (Haney 2005). Dara's school anxiety might have been made even more intense by marijuana's tendency to impair focus and concentration, which can make academic work feel almost impossible.

With regard to a primary anxiety disorder, it is useful to recall that anxiety disorders—like many psychiatric disorders—often make their first appearance during adolescence, and approximately 15%–20% of adolescents with SUDs have a co-occurring anxiety disorder (O'Neil et al. 2011). It is possible, therefore, that Dara's psychiatric symptoms began during heavy cannabis use but that they reflect a primary psychiatric disorder. Definitive diagnoses in adolescents must often be deferred until the patient has been abstinent for weeks or months.

## Screening and Assessment

All adolescents who come to psychiatric attention should be specifically screened for substance use. Adolescent-specific screening instruments can be helpful. For example, CRAFFT, a simple screening tool designed to identify adolescent substance use, can be used. CRAFFT is a mnemonic for six yes/no questions that probe whether an adolescent has: driven or been driven in a **C**AR while using drugs or alcohol, used drugs or alcohol to **R**ELAX, used **A**LONE, **F**ORGOTTEN what happened (blacked out) while using, been told by FAMILY or FRIENDS to cut down, or gotten in TROUBLE while using drugs or alcohol (Knight et al. 1999). If a patient screens positive, a more detailed history should be obtained. For example, it can be helpful to know which substances have been used and used when, in what quantity, with whom, how frequently, and with what results. Collateral information can be helpful, particularly since adolescents often underreport the amount, frequency, and consequences of use. Parents should be interviewed about the adolescent's use as well as about family history of psychiatric and substance use disorders, as well as about current patterns of substance use by other members of the household. A functional analysis, which explores the antecedents and consequences of the adolescent's substance use, should be carried out (Bukstein et al. 2005). It can also be helpful to explore the adolescent's own view of a potential substance problem, as well as any attempts the adolescent has made to address the perceived problem.

To be diagnosed with a substance use *disorder,* a patient must demonstrate impairment in one or more domains of his or her life, such as school, extracurricular, family and peer relationships, physical health, and psychiatric health (Bukstein et al. 2005). Dara's marijuana use appears to have affected many aspects of her life. Even if she does not herself perceive a problem, her substance use warrants a diagnosis of a SUD. Further evaluation would also address whether she has an alcohol use disorder and a tobacco use disorder. If an adolescent is using substances but is not experiencing impairment, he or she can be considered to be at high risk for a disorder and can—and likely should—still be treated.

# Treatment

The first step in determining a treatment plan is to address safety. Is the patient intoxicated at the time of assessment? Is the patient using a substance that could cause a dangerous withdrawal if stopped abruptly, such as alcohol, barbiturates, or benzodiazepines? Is the patient at risk of lethal overdose, which could occur with opioids, for example? In Dara's case, cannabis has not caused physiologically dangerous intoxication or withdrawal. Assuming her more dangerous behaviors (subway jumping, unprotected sex) are not deemed to be acutely life threatening, she can be treated initially as an outpatient. However, if safety is a concern, inpatient hospitalization would be the essential first step in treatment.

Once safety is assured, the next step is to determine whether a harm-reduction or abstinence-based approach is most realistic for the patient. Whereas with adult patients, it is primarily the patient's degree of motivation that determines this, with adolescents, the parents or court may play a role as well. Are the parents/guardians willing to participate actively in the treatment process, as is required in a contingency management treatment (see below)? Or do they feel overwhelmed and unable to set limits for their child, such that an inpatient or residential setting would be more effective? Outpatient treatment can be described along an intensity continuum from office-based care to IOP (intensive outpatient) to PHP (partial hospitalization program). The next level of intensity would be residential treatment, followed by inpatient treatment with medical detoxification as necessary (i.e., for alcohol, opioids, or benzodiazepines).

In Dara's case, her parents are highly motivated, as is Dara herself, to address the symptoms of inattention and anxiety. While her parents are generally in favor of their child's long-term abstinence, it is not clear whether Dara herself is willing to agree to pursue abstinence. This is typical of adolescents, who have difficulty conceptualizing a long life without substances. The dissonance between parents' and adolescents' treatment goals is common, and can usually be navigated clinically.

## Psychosocial Interventions

While motivational interviewing (MI), motivational enhancement therapy (MET), 12-step group treatment, and cognitive-behavioral therapy (CBT) are all as applicable to the adolescent patient as they are to the adult (with some modifications for age-appropriateness), there are three psychosocial interventions that are of particular utility in the adolescent population.

### Contingency Management

Contingency management is a treatment system created together by the clinician, parents, adolescent, and other stakeholders (school administrators, sports coaches, court officials) to determine tangible rewards for abstinence or other desired behaviors. In Dara's case, a contingency could be set up in which Dara would receive $25 for every consecutive negative weekly urine test, which she could put toward a specific purchase. Contingency management can be an effective element of overall treatment for an adolescent because the parents and other stakeholders are actively involved in motivating the recovery. Providing a tangible benefit can be particularly useful for adolescents in the early phases of recovery, since they may not yet appreciate an intrinsic value in abstaining.

## Family Therapies

There are several types of evidence-based family therapies that are well-suited to address the interpersonal dynamics that arise around an adolescent substance user. Multidimensional family therapy (MDFT) consists of individual patient sessions and family sessions that can be held in the home, clinic, school, or court setting and aim to mitigate the influences that lead the adolescent to use substances (National Institute on Drug Abuse 2012).

Brief strategic family therapy (BSFT) targets family interactions that are thought to exacerbate or maintain adolescent substance use and can be flexibly used in outpatient, residential, and social services settings (National Institute on Drug Abuse 2012).

Functional family therapy (FFT) is similar to MDFT and BSFT in that it targets family dynamics that promote substance use in the adolescent, but it is unique in that every session includes the adolescent and at least one family member. FFT is a behavioral treatment that employs contingency management for family members as well as the adolescent, behavioral contracts, and other behavioral interventions to enhance motivation for change throughout the entire family system (National Institute on Drug Abuse 2012).

## CRAFT

Community Reinforcement Approach and Family Treatment (CRAFT), not to be confused with the CRAFFT screening tool discussed above, is a "unilateral" treatment in that it can be used when the individual with the substance use problem (the adolescent) is not himself or herself engaging in treatment. CRAFT is designed to help a significant other (usually a parent) reduce the adolescent's substance use, engage him or her in treatment, and improve the psychosocial well-being of the parent and family (Foote and Wilkens 2014; http://the20minuteguide.com). It teaches parents how to respond to substance use behaviors by reinforcing positive (i.e., non–substance use) behaviors, withdrawing reinforcers for negative (i.e., substance use) behaviors, and allowing natural consequences to occur. Reinforcers should be easy to provide and feel comfortable for the parents to provide or withdraw. Natural consequences should be safe and therefore feel tolerable to the parent. In Dara's case, an example of a natural consequence would be letting her sleep through her Saturday drama club rehearsal rather than waking her so that she would not miss it. Such a consequence would feel safer and more comfortable to Dara's parents than, for example, letting her sleep through the SAT, but would still demonstrate to her the negative outcomes associated with her substance use. CRAFT also teaches parents how to communicate more effectively with the adolescent, and how to motivate the adolescent into treatment (Foote and Wilkens 2014; http://the20minuteguide.com).

Although CRAFT is designed to be unilateral, it can still be useful when the adolescent *is* engaged in treatment: as we will see, Dara *does* commit to treatment, but her parents certainly benefit from learning, with the help of the psychiatrist, how to better communicate with Dara, and how to use reinforcers to encourage non-substance-using behavior and discourage use behavior.

## PHARMACOLOGICAL INTERVENTIONS

There are no U.S. Food and Drug Administration (FDA)–approved medications for the treatment of cannabis use disorder. The FDA-approved medications for other substance use disorders, such as naltrexone for alcohol or opioid use disorders, disulfiram for alcohol use disorder, or buprenorphine and methadone for opioid use disorders, are not approved for patients under the age of 18. These medications can be used off-label after the failure of psychosocial interventions, though off-label use in minors requires informed consent from the patient and parents.

Comorbidity is common in adolescent substance use. Selective serotonin reuptake inhibitors (SSRIs) for unipolar depression and anxiety, stimulants for ADHD, mood stabilizers for bipolar depression and mania, and antipsychotics for psychotic disorders are all appropriate for use in adolescents.

# Dara's Treatment

Dara's case illustrates how several of the treatment modalities discussed above can be combined in a comprehensive treatment.

Feedback to the patient and parents took place over several meetings. At first, during individual meetings with Dara, the psychiatrist validated her anxiety about academic performance and college admissions and her desire to seek relaxation by spending time with her friends and using cannabis. The psychiatrist suggested that it was possible that her cannabis use, though intended to help her anxiety and insomnia, may be making them worse. He also posited that cannabis was producing cognitive effects that were impairing her academic performance. Dara was at first reluctant to disclose information about her cannabis use and its effects to her parents, but ultimately agreed to do so, stating that it was "their fault [she was] a drug addict" because they put so much pressure on her to "over-achieve."

In a family meeting with the psychiatrist, Dara disclosed to her parents details about her cannabis use, including her frequency of use and her reasons for using. She explained that it helped relieve anxiety but that she was at the same time afraid of getting caught, being expelled from school, and not getting into the right college.

The psychiatrist shared the following working diagnostic formulation with Dara and her family: 1) cannabis use disorder, severe and 2) substance-induced anxiety disorder vs. adjustment disorder with anxiety vs. generalized anxiety disorder.

He explained that ADHD was ruled out based on clinical history and rating scales, and thus did not recommend stimulant medication, neuropsychological testing, or extended time on tests.

Her parents' initial response was anger. Psychoeducation and supportive psychotherapy by the psychiatrist during that session and in subsequent sessions allowed the parents to ally with Dara to come up with a collaborative treatment plan that consisted of

1. Weekly visits to the psychiatrist for therapy and medication management.
2. Weekly urine drug testing at the psychiatrist's office.
3. Contingency management with parents that included twice-monthly family sessions based on CRAFT principles.

For the first 3 weeks of treatment, Dara's qualitative urine tests were positive for cannabis. She reported that in trying to reduce use by not smoking during lunch or before bed, she felt tremulous, diaphoretic, and irritable and had constant headaches. For this reason, she continued to use cannabis after school and on weekends with her boyfriend. The psychiatrist used MET and started escitalopram, increasing the dose from 2.5 mg to 5 mg to 10 mg to 15 mg daily. Dara remained ambivalent about stopping her cannabis use altogether into week 5 of treatment, but ultimately responded to the MET along with a contingency set up by her parents by which she would earn $25 toward an expensive designer handbag she wanted. She would receive $25 for every *consecutive* week of negative urine tests, with an interceding positive week reducing her back to $0.

At week 7, Dara had her first negative urine test result and began reporting feeling less anxious, which she and her psychiatrist agreed was likely due to a combination of cannabis cessation and the effects of the escitalopram. She tested positive for cannabis at week 12, explaining that she had smoked once in the context of breaking up with her boyfriend the previous weekend. She added that she could no longer tolerate being around "such a stoner." She described feeling guilty for relapsing and angry that she had to start back at $0 toward the handbag. After 10 consecutive weeks of negative urine tests, the testing was reduced to every other week, and psychotherapy shifted from being focused mostly on MET to a broader focus on coping with anxiety. By the end of eleventh grade, Dara had improved her grades to all B's and had earned her handbag. In June, she took the SAT and was able to complete all sections within the allotted time.

Throughout the course of treatment, Dara's parents accompanied her to appointments every 2 weeks. The psychiatrist taught Dara and her parents how to communicate more effectively, particularly around academic expectations and substance use. For example, these communication techniques helped Dara explain to her parents that she got anxious when they applied academic pressure by getting angry about her grades, while her parents were able to effectively explain that though they did sometimes react angrily, they were concerned about her well-being and not whether she would attend the "right" college.

Dara continued taking escitalopram for the remainder of high school. During twelfth grade, she had monthly urine tests with the psychiatrist, who referred her for CBT with a psychologist to address anxiety that continued to be an episodic problem.

# Conclusion

The assessment and treatment of adolescents with substance use disorders is different from that in adults. First, the entire family ecosystem must be involved; second, the adolescent brain's unique developmental characteristics must be considered; and third, confidentiality issues must be addressed in an adolescent-specific manner. SUDs in adolescents can masquerade as or exacerbate other primary psychiatric disorders, which should be assessed and treated simultaneously. The best-studied treatments for adolescent SUDs are psychosocial in nature and involve the patient's family and/or other social framework.

## KEY POINTS

- Adolescence is a uniquely vulnerable developmental period with regard to substance use disorders (SUDs) because of an imbalance of activity in the brain reward system versus cognitive control and risk avoidance ("bottom up" drives overwhelm "top down" controls).

- All adolescents should be screened for substance use and assessed for SUDs if they screen positive.

- Treatment of the adolescent substance user is different from that of the adult in that it usually involves the entire family.
- Contingency management, family therapy, and CRAFT are effective psychosocial interventions for adolescent SUDs.
- Co-occurring psychiatric disorders, which are the norm rather than the exception, should be treated psychosocially and/or pharmacologically in conjunction with substance use treatment.

# Questions

1. A 15-year-old patient presents to the emergency room in a post-ictal state after a witnessed seizure with a urine toxicology positive for benzodiazepines. The first step in management is

    A. Refer to an outpatient clinic for a substance abuse evaluation.
    B. Call parents and provide them with a list of 12-step groups in the area that are geared toward adolescents and young adults.
    C. Admit to the neurology service for epilepsy workup.
    D. Observe in emergency department, checking vital signs frequently, and attempt to obtain collateral history from parents and/or peers.

2. Which of the following is a primary reason adolescence is a developmentally vulnerable period with regard to the development of substance use problems?

    A. The brain continues to develop until the mid-twenties.
    B. The "top-down" controls provided by the prefrontal cortex cannot be overruled by the "bottom-up" force of the reward system in adolescents.
    C. The risk-avoidance mechanism of the amygdala cannot be overridden by the reward-seeking mechanism of the ventral striatum.
    D. The adolescent brain has more opioid receptors than the adult brain because they have not yet been fully pruned.

3. The following approach is best for maintaining an adolescent's request for confidentiality while also maintaining her safety with regard to substance use:

A. Advise the adolescent that if she does not disclose her use to the parent, the clinician will do so.

B. Advise the adolescent that confidentiality will be maintained, no matter what, so the adolescent should feel secure sharing anything with the clinician.

C. Advise the adolescent that engaging her parents in treatment will make it most effective, such that some information that the adolescent discloses to the clinician may be metabolized into treatment recommendations that are given to the parents.

D. Advise the adolescent that confidentiality will only be breached if safety becomes an issue, and that any substance use behaviors in an adolescent are inherently unsafe.

# References

Buckner JD, Schmidt NB: Marijuana effect expectancies: relations to social anxiety and cannabis use problems. Addict Behav 33:1477–1483, 2008 18694625

Bukstein OG, Bernet W, Arnold V, et al; Work Group on Quality Issues: Practice parameter for the assessment and treatment of children and adolescents with substance use disorders. J Am Acad Child Adolesc Psychiatry 44(6):609–621, 2005 15908844

Casey BJ, Jones RM: Neurobiology of the adolescent brain and behavior: implications for substance use disorders. J Am Acad Child Adolesc Psychiatry 49(12):1189–1201, quiz 1285, 2010 21093769

Ernst M: The triadic model perspective for the study of adolescent motivated behavior. Brain Cogn 89:104–111, 2014 24556507

Foote J, Wilkens C: Beyond Addiction. New York, Scribner, 2014

Haney M: The marijuana withdrawal syndrome: diagnosis and treatment. Curr Psychiatry Rep 7(5):360–366, 2005 16216154

Jacobus J, Bava S, Cohen-Zion M, et al: Functional consequences of marijuana use in adolescents. Pharmacol Biochem Behav 92(4):559–565, 2009 19348837

Knight JR, Shrier LA, Bravender TD, et al: A new brief screen for adolescent substance abuse. Arch Pediatr Adolesc Med 153(6):591–596, 1999 10357299

Medina KL, Hanson KL, Schweinsburg AD, et al: Neuropsychological functioning in adolescent marijuana users: subtle deficits detectable after a month of abstinence. J Int Neuropsychol Soc 13(5):807–820, 2007 17697412

National Institute on Drug Abuse: Principles of Drug Addiction Treatment: A Research-Based Guide, 3rd Edition. December 2012. Available at: https://www.drugabuse.gov/publications/principles-drug-addiction-treatment-research-based-guide-third-edition/evidence-based-approaches-to-drug-addiction-treatment/behavioral-6. Accessed February 7, 2017.

O'Neil KA, Conner BT, Kendall PC: Internalizing disorders and substance use disorders in youth: comorbidity, risk, temporal order, and implications for intervention. Clin Psychol Rev 31(1):104–112, 2011 20817371

Rosner R: The Clinical Handbook of Adolescent Addiction. West Sussex, UK, Wiley, 2013, pp 83, 337, 340

Tau GZ, Peterson BS: Normal development of brain circuits. Neuropsychopharmacology 35(1):147–168, 2010 19794405

Wolraich ML, Hannah JN, Baumgaertel A, Feurer ID: Examination of DSM-IV criteria for attention deficit/hyperactivity disorder in a county-wide sample. J Dev Behav Pediatr 19(3):162–168, 1998 9648041

# 16

# GERIATRICS

*Caitlin Snow, M.D.*

The transition from middle to old age tends to be accompanied by reduced rates of depression, anxiety, and substance use. At the same time, the elderly tend to develop medical illnesses that diminish well-being and complicate psychiatric diagnosis and treatment. Further, the "baby boom" generation is entering old age, and, as has been the case throughout their lives, they bring with them a large demographic impact. For one thing, there are many of them: the population of U.S. adults age 65 and older is expected to almost double within 20 years (from 40.3 million in 2010 to a projected 72.1 million in 2030) (Institute of Medicine 2012). In addition, substance use disorders are far more prevalent among baby boomers than among preceding generations (Gfroerer et al. 2003). Although common, substance abuse may not manifest itself in the same ways as it does in younger populations, leading substance use disorders (SUDs) among older adults to be coined an "invisible epidemic" (Blow 1998).

This chapter will emphasize ways that older people with co-occurring psychiatric and substance use disorders differ from their younger counterparts. This perspective is especially important given that there are insufficient numbers of specialists who have been trained to meet the need of this population (Institute of Medicine 2012). The chapter begins with a case of a man whose co-occurring disorders (CODs) are fairly common within the geriatric population.

## Clinical Case

William is a 70-year-old man with no formal psychiatric history who presents for a psychiatric evaluation accompanied by his adult daughter. Concerned her father has looked "out of it" and "unhappy" for the prior 6 months, she had already taken him to a neurologist, who concluded that he did not have Alzheimer's disease or some other neurocognitive disorder. She had accepted a referral to a psychopharmacologist, who diagnosed a depression and began an antidepressant medication. Two months later William's symptoms had not improved, and so his daughter was bringing him in for a second psychiatric opinion.

William divorced in his early 50s and retired from his job in advertising sales at age 65. He lives alone in a suburban community and denies religious affiliation. He has a medical history of hypertension, hyperlipidemia, gastroesophageal reflux disease, diabetes mellitus type II, and chronic lower back pain. For the past decade, William has been taking stable doses of a beta-blocker, prophylactic aspirin, a statin, a proton pump inhibitor, a hypoglycemic agent, and a short-acting opioid as needed. He reports that he is adherent with all of his medications, but notes that for the past several weeks he has increased the frequency of his opioid use due to an exacerbation of chronic pain. William and his daughter report that he has always been an outgoing, gregarious man who continues to talk to friends even if he "doesn't feel like it." He says he does not miss working and does not feel especially lonely, but that he does not seem to be enjoying his many hobbies as much as he thought he should.

William specifically denies a problem with alcohol and drugs, including the opioid. He does say he likes a "nightcap," which he quantifies as two 1.5 oz. shots of whiskey. This had been his routine for his adult life and had caused him "no problems." Over the past several months, William reports, he has been drinking an additional shot or two of whiskey nightly in an effort to reduce his back pain and fall asleep. He also says he "very rarely" uses some of his daughter's lorazepam to help him sleep. He reports drinking approximately five shots of whiskey while socializing with friends, a pattern that he describes as constant for decades. He does not feel concerned by his alcohol consumption and has made no effort to cut down. When asked if he has ever felt annoyed by someone inquiring about his alcohol consumption, he responds, "Sure, my daughter is annoying that way." He scores a 5 out of 10 on the SMAST-G rating scale. He denies tobacco and illicit drug use.

On exam, William appears well dressed and cooperative. He says he is "doing fine" overall but reports difficulty sleeping with middle and late insomnia, low energy, and diminished motivation. He states that he naps frequently during the day because of boredom and daytime fatigue. He acknowledges that his mood has been "a little down," but he minimizes his daughter's concern that he is depressed and believes that this is an appropriate emotional response to his life circumstances. Although he has made less effort to socialize with peers, he continues to derive social support from his weekly "whiskey and poker" nights. On review of physical symptoms, he endorses several days of black tarry stools that resolved without intervention, episodic lightheadedness when standing, and chronic lower back pain. He dismisses all of these complaints as "old man problems."

# Discussion

William was brought for a psychiatric evaluation because his daughter noticed that he seemed "out of it" and "unhappy." Her first concern had been dementia, but the neurologist did not find a neurocognitive disorder. Her next concern was depression, which could be consistent with his reports of unhappiness, insomnia, low energy, and diminished motivation. The first psychiatrist did diagnose a depression and started an antidepressant medication. William and his daughter were presenting for a second opinion when the antidepressant medication had not improved his mood after 2 months. The lack of effect of the antidepressant might indicate the need for a medication switch or an additional treatment (e.g., psychotherapy or a psychosocial program). The lack of effect should also remind the clinician to look for additional diagnoses.

Could an alcohol use disorder be contributing to William's unhappiness, insomnia, anergia, diminished motivation, and appearance of being "out of it"? William does not think so, seeming to view his alcohol use as long-standing and without complications. Nevertheless, his daily alcohol use seems to have increased from 3 to 6 ounces in recent months, and he reports drinking 5 drinks (7.5 ounces) when he goes out with his friends each week. As is the case with younger drinkers, older people may minimize their alcohol use, and so it is certainly possible that William's intake is significantly greater than his initial report. Even if we accept his alcohol estimate, his use probably meets the National Institute on Alcohol Abuse and Alcoholism definitions for both "heavy drinking" and "binge drinking." William is likely to receive recommendations to cut down his alcohol consumption with skepticism. For the clinical interaction to have relevance with a patient like William, it will be useful to be able to discuss some of the epidemiological, physiological, and psychiatric realities that will be addressed in this chapter.

It will also be useful for the clinician to pay attention to William's report that he has recently increased his use of opioids to treat his chronic low back pain. Alcohol and opioids can either contribute to a major depression or be—by themselves—the core contributor to an array of psychiatric symptoms, including all of the symptoms that have reduced William's quality of life.

*Clinicians are often slow to diagnose substance use disorders in the elderly,* frequently because of inappropriate assumptions. Although there is an overall decline in illicit substance abuse as people age, SUDs are still common in the elderly. Further, even the stable use of alcohol or a prescribed medication can become problematic as people age and their tolerance declines. Some clinicians do not pursue the possibility of a SUD because they anticipate that the elderly cannot change their behaviors, or that "they deserve their small pleasures," or that they would be offended by being accused of being an alcoholic or drug addict (Blow 1998). While there may be some truth to each of these concerns, tactful exploration and treatment of a substance use disorder in the elderly can be life changing.

*Brief, low-cost, and expedient standardized screening tools have been adapted for the geriatric population.* The most frequently used tools to screen for at-risk alcohol use in older adults are the CAGE questionnaire (Mayfield et al. 1974), the Short Michigan Alcoholism Screening Test—Geriatric Version (SMAST-G; Naegle 2008) (Table 16–1), and the Alcohol Use Disorders Identification Test (AUDIT; Bush et al. 1998). The threshold for the CAGE questionnaire is typically lowered to one positive response in older adults as the trigger for further exploration. In the case of William, he screened positive by indicating that he felt annoyed by his daughter's criticism of his drinking, thereby warranting further evaluation. William's SMAST-G screen was also positive, given that a score of

---

**TABLE 16–1.** **Short Michigan Alcoholism Screening Test—Geriatric Version (SMAST-G)**

---

Please answer Yes or No to the following questions:

1. When talking with others, do you ever underestimate how much you drink?
2. After a few drinks, have you sometimes not eaten or been able to skip a meal because you didn't feel hungry?
3. Does having a few drinks help decrease your shakiness or tremors?
4. Does alcohol sometimes make it hard for you to remember parts of the day or night?
5. Do you usually take a drink to calm your nerves?
6. Do you drink to take your mind off your problems?
7. Have you ever increased your drinking after experiencing a loss in your life?
8. Has a doctor or nurse ever said they were worried or concerned about your drinking?
9. Have you ever made rules to manage your drinking?
10. When you feel lonely, does having a drink help?

---

SCORING: Score 1 point for each "yes" answer and total the responses; 2+ points are indicative of an alcohol problem.

---

*Source.* Adapted from Naegle 2008.

---

2+ indicates an alcohol problem that warrants a brief intervention. Of note, there is evidence that CAGE and SMAST-G detect different aspects of problem drinking in older adults, suggesting there is benefit in combining the screening measures so as to increase sensitivity (Moore et al. 2002).

*Alcohol use disorders are common in older adults.* Prevalence estimates vary across settings and based on diagnostic criteria. According to the 2012 National Survey on Drug Use and Health, 41.2% of adults age 65 and older had consumed alcohol in the past month, with 8.2% reporting binge use, which is defined as five or more drinks on any one occasion. Two percent of people over 65 report heavy use, which is defined as five or more drinks on each of five or more occasions (Substance Abuse and Mental Health Services Administration 2013) (Table 16–2). Estimated rates of alcohol use are higher in clinical settings than in community samples and are particularly high in health care–seeking populations (Blow et al. 2007; Oslin and Mavandadi 2013). Since clinicians are, by

---

**TABLE 16–2.  Percent alcohol usage in past month, age 65 and older**

| | |
|---|---|
| Current alcohol use | 41.2% |
| Binge use (5+ drinks on any one occasion) | 8.2% |
| Heavy alcohol use (5+ drinks on each of 5 or more occasions in the prior 30 days) | 2.0% |
| Tobacco use | 10.0% |
| Illicit drug use | 1.3% |

*Source.*   Simoni-Wasila and Yang 2006.

---

definition, seeing "health care–seeking" patients, they should expect that a significant percentage of their patients have a SUD.

When we are trying to identify which patients are more likely to have an alcohol use disorder, it is useful to recall that older men have higher rates of problematic alcohol use, as do those who are divorced or widowed, who lack a religious affiliation, and who are in the young-old age group (e.g., ages 65–74). Age-related losses in social and occupational domains, as well as medical and psychiatric comorbidity, have also been shown to be associated with late-life drinking problems (Oslin and Mavandadi 2013). In many ways, William is typical of an individual at risk for developing an alcohol use disorder: he is divorced, medically ill, and nonreligious and belongs to the young-old age group.

*The use of prescription and over-the-counter drugs has increased in older adults,* thereby exacerbating the risks of drug-drug interactions and drug misuse (Oslin and Mavandadi 2013). The rate of prescription drug misuse in older women is estimated to be 11%, which is higher than the rate observed in older men. Rates are particularly high in women who are divorced or widowed and of lower socioeconomic status. Co-occurring psychiatric diagnoses increase the risk of prescription drug abuse in both men and women (Simoni-Wasila and Yang 2006). Given William's chronic pain and opioid use, he should be closely monitored for misuse potential as well as medication interactions.

*Older adults are physiologically more vulnerable to the deleterious effects of alcohol, illicit substances, and over-the-counter and prescription drugs* (Gambert and Katsoyannis 1995). Contributing factors include a decrease in lean body mass and total water volume relative to total fat volume, reduced efficiency of metabolic enzymes such as alcohol dehydrogenase in the gastric mucosa and liver, decreased hepatic and renal size, decreased hepatic and renal blood flow, and increased sensitivity of the central nervous system. As in the case of William, age-related changes will cause equivalent amounts of alcohol and opiates to result in a higher blood alcohol concentration and an enhanced effect of opiates. This can result in the type of nonspecific physical and cognitive symptoms that William presented with, such as daytime fatigue, sleep disturbance, low mood, and cognitive slowing.

Alcohol can lead directly to health problems as well as neuropsychiatric symptoms such as insomnia, mood, and memory problems (Gambert and Katsoyannis 1995). Further, problematic alcohol use has been shown to trigger and worsen diabetes, cardiovascular disease, liver disease, and a variety of cancers. Alcohol is also associated with the development of neurocognitive disorders (Oslin and Mavandadi 2013). Even in someone without a SUD, occasional intoxication greatly increases the risk of falls, which lead to such problems as hip fractures, which commonly worsen the morbidity and mortality in the elderly. Symptomatic alcohol withdrawal (including delirium tremens) is common in situations where the alcohol use disorder is not elicited.

*Older adults are often prescribed multiple medications with the potential for complicating interactions.* For example, William is apparently prescribed a beta-blocker, prophylactic aspirin, a statin, a proton pump inhibitor, a hypoglycemic agent, and a short-acting opioid. We do not know the names of these six prescribed medications, but drug-drug interactions are a not-uncommon cause for a reduced quality of life in older people.

*Alcohol also affects the metabolism of other drugs.* As a general rule, acute alcohol intoxication inhibits the cytochrome P450 system and can thereby prolong the half-life of some prescribed medications. In contrast, chronic alcohol ingestion causes enzymatic induction of the cytochrome P450 system and can lead to the rapid metabolism and diminished drug efficacy of prescribed medications. Common medication interactions with alcohol that were highlighted in the clinical case of William are summarized in Table 16–3.

William admits to occasionally treating his insomnia with his daughter's lorazepam. Medication diversion is common among the elderly, and it is often not spontaneously mentioned. Older adults are especially prone to common benzodiazepine effects, such as memory impairment, sedation, falls, and motor vehicle accidents (Charlson et al. 2009). Benzodiazepines are often prescribed to older adults despite these risks, sometimes because the patient has been taking them for years and "can't sleep with anything else." We do not know the extent of William's use of lorazepam, but even modest use would intensify alcohol-related intoxication, dependence, and withdrawal.

*Older adults who engage in substance abuse treatment have better attendance and adherence when compared with their younger counterparts and have comparable, and possibly better, outcomes.* Evidence also indicates that sub-

**TABLE 16–3.** Common medication interactions with alcohol

| Medication class | Effects | Clinical case notes |
| --- | --- | --- |
| Beta-blockers | Increased hypotension | May account for dizziness when standing |
| NSAIDs (*aspirin) | Increased risk of gastrointestinal bleeding<br>*Decreased gastric alcohol dehydrogenase activity | May account for black tarry stools<br>*Impaired first-pass metabolism<br>Equivalent amounts of alcohol lead to higher blood alcohol concentration |
| Proton pump inhibitors | Decreased gastric alcohol dehydrogenase activity | Impaired first-pass metabolism<br>Equivalent amounts of alcohol lead to higher blood alcohol concentration |
| Statins | Increased hepatic toxicity | Should monitor with routine blood work |
| Hypoglycemic agents (*metformin) | Hypoglycemia<br>*Increased risk of lactic acidosis | Could account for weakness, fatigue, and irritability |
| Opioids | Increased sedative effect and hypotension | May account for fatigue, low energy, and dizziness when standing |

stance abuse treatment is more effective when it addresses issues relevant to the older age group and when the treatment is delivered in an integrated setting rather than a specialty clinic (Oslin and Mavandadi 2013).

Brief psychosocial interventions have been shown to be efficient and cost effective and to significantly diminish alcohol, illicit drug, and medication misuse across a variety of settings among older adults (Oslin and Mavandadi 2013). Typical characteristics of these brief interventions include psychoeducation, motivational interviewing, and referral to more intensive treatments on an as-needed basis. A brief intervention would be useful to employ when treating a patient similar to William.

Twelve-step peer support programs and self-help groups have mixed results in older adults. Although rates of attendance are similar across age groups, older adults may have lower levels of engagement when compared with their younger counterparts (Satre et al. 2004). Research also suggests that older adults attend formal rehab programs at lower rates and engage at lower levels when compared with their younger counterparts (Satre et al. 2004). These differences may be due to perceived stigma, discomfort with the mixed-age and group setting, and logistical barriers.

*Medication treatments for alcohol use disorders in older adults are not thoroughly studied.* Acamprosate may be the most effective medication to reduce alcohol use, but it has not been adequately studied in an older population (Barrick and Connors 2002). Of note, acamprosate is excreted unmetabolized, so it can be considered in patients with hepatic dysfunction, although it should be used with caution in patients with renal impairment.

Naltrexone is the best studied, but evidence for its use has been modest and inconsistent. Interestingly, in a study of late-life depression complicated by alcohol dependence, there was no difference between naltrexone and placebo in remission of either depression or the alcohol use disorder. The study did demonstrate, however, that alcohol relapse predicted a poor response to the antidepressant (Oslin 2005). This underscores the importance of identifying and treating all co-occurring substance and psychiatric illnesses that are present in older individuals like William. Of note, an additional limitation to the use of naltrexone in this patient population is that, as in the case study, many older adults have chronic pain and naltrexone can block the effect of prescribed opiate pain medications.

Disulfiram, which inhibits alcohol dehydrogenase, has not been shown to be effective and is avoided in older adults because of the risk of serious side effects, including cardiovascular compromise.

# Conclusion

Substance use disorders are a growing health problem in the geriatric population. The case of William illustrates a common presentation of an older adult with an alcohol use disorder. SUDs are underdiagnosed and undertreated despite the availability of effective interventions. Treatment of an individual like William should ideally address all co-occurring medical and psychiatric issues with psychosocial and pharmacological treatment options as indicated.

## KEY POINTS

- Substance use disorders (SUDs) among older adults remain underdetected and undertreated despite increasing prevalence.

- Diagnostic thresholds for SUDs in older adults have been lowered to reflect the increased vulnerability of this patient population due to age-related physiological changes, medical comorbidity, and medication interactions.

- Co-occurring medical, neurological, and psychiatric conditions are common and may impact treatment outcomes.

- A variety of treatments for SUDs have been shown to be effective among older adults, and older adults who engage in treatment have better adherence when compared with their younger counterparts.

- Age-specific treatment and an integrated care setting have been shown to improve attendance and engagement in treatment in older adults.

- There is modest but inconsistent support for the role of pharmacotherapy in the treatment of SUDs in older adults.

# Questions

1. Which of the following statements is *true* regarding substance use disorders (SUDs) in older adults?

   A. Demographic trends suggest a decreasing prevalence of SUDs in older adults in the coming decade.

B. Older men have not been shown to have higher rates of alcohol and psychoactive substance problems when compared with older women.

C. Overall alcohol use increases with age.

D. Older adults who engage in treatment have worse adherence when compared with their younger counterparts.

2. Which of the following statements is *true* regarding the diagnosis of SUDs in older adults?

A. SUDs in older adults are underdetected and underdiagnosed.

B. With age, referrals for treatment of SUDs are less likely to come from primary care settings and more likely to come from the criminal justice system.

C. Guidelines recommend the same level of alcohol consumption in older adults and the same thresholds to diagnose problematic drinking.

D. There are no validated screening tools for alcohol use disorder that have been specifically adapted for the geriatric population.

3. Which of the following characteristics of treatment for SUDs are positively correlated with engagement and response in older adults?

A. Mixed-age treatment and specialty care setting.

B. Age-specific treatment and specialty care setting.

C. Mixed-age treatment and integrated care setting.

D. Age-specific treatment and integrated care setting.

# References

Barrick C, Connors GJ: Relapse prevention and maintaining abstinence in older adults with alcohol-use disorders. Drugs Aging 19(8):583–594, 2002 12207552

Blow FC: Substance Abuse Among Older Adults: An Invisible Epidemic. Treatment Improvement Protocol (TIP) Series, No 26 (DHHS Publ No SMA-98–3179). Rockville, MD, Substance Abuse and Mental Health Services Administration, 1998

Blow FC, Serras AM, Barry KL: Late-life depression and alcoholism. Curr Psychiatry Rep 9(1):14–19, 2007 17257508

Bush K, Kivlahan DR, McDonell MB, et al: The AUDIT alcohol consumption questions (AUDIT-C): an effective brief screening test for problem drinking. Arch Intern Med 158(16):1789–1795, 1998 9738608

Charlson F, Degenhardt L, McLaren J, et al: A systematic review of research examining benzodiazepine-related mortality. Pharmacoepidemiol Drug Saf 18(2):93–103, 2009 19125401

Gambert SR, Katsoyannis KK: Alcohol-related medical disorders of older heavy drinkers, in Alcohol and Aging. Edited by Beresford TP, Gomberg E. New York, Oxford University Press, 1995, pp 70–81

Gfroerer J, Penne M, Pemberton M, Folsom R: Substance abuse treatment need among older adults in 2020: the impact of the aging baby-boom cohort. Drug Alcohol Depend 69(2):127–135, 2003 12609694

Institute of Medicine: The Mental Health and Substance Use Workforce for Older Adults: In Whose Hands? Washington, DC, National Academy of Sciences, 2012

Mayfield D, McLeod G, Hall P: The CAGE questionnaire: validation of a new alcoholism screening instrument. Am J Psychiatry 131(10):1121–1123, 1974 4416585

Moore AA, Seeman T, Morgenstern H, et al: Are there differences between older persons who screen positive on the CAGE questionnaire and the Short Michigan Alcoholism Screening Test-Geriatric Version? J Am Geriatr Soc 50(5):858–862, 2002 12028172

Naegle MA: Screening for alcohol use and misuse in older adults: using the Short Michigan Alcoholism Screening Test—Geriatric Version. Am J Nurs 108(11):50–58, quiz 58–59, 2008 18946267

Oslin DW: Treatment of late-life depression complicated by alcohol dependence. Am J Geriatr Psychiatry 13(6):491–500, 2005 15956269

Oslin DW, Mavandadi S: Alcohol and drug problems, in Clinical Manual of Geriatric Psychiatry. Edited by Thakur ME, Blazer DG, Steffens DC. Washington, DC, American Psychiatric Association, 2013, pp 211–234

Satre DD, Mertens JR, Areán PA, et al: Five-year alcohol and drug treatment outcomes of older adults versus middle-aged and younger adults in a managed care program. Addiction 99(10):1286–1297, 2004 15369567

Simoni-Wastila L, Yang HK: Psychoactive drug abuse in older adults. Am J Geriatr Pharmacother 4(4):380–394, 2006 17296542

Substance Abuse and Mental Health Services Administration: Results from the 2012 National Survey on Drug Use and Health: Summary of National Findings, NSDUH Series H-46 (HHS Publ No SMA-13–4795). Rockville, MD, Substance Abuse and Mental Health Services Administration, 2013

# 17

# LGBTQ POPULATION

### Eric Yarbrough, M.D.

People who are members of stigmatized populations tend to receive suboptimal psychiatric care. Marginalized and sometimes targeted by people and institutions within their community, they may have increased rates of co-occurring psychiatric and substance use disorders but reduced access to mental health services. They may also be wary of seeking care from clinicians who might share the broader cultural bias. These realities have certainly been true for members of the lesbian, gay, bisexual, transgender, and queer or questioning (LGBTQ) population. Despite significant advances in regard to broad cultural acceptance, members of the LGBTQ community continue to face community criticism, governmental efforts to allow conversion therapy, and mental health professionals who may have been trained to view their identity and/or sexual orientation as aberrant and pathological. Aware of the many potential biases, people in desperate need may be wary of seeking psychiatric help.

To effectively treat co-occurring disorders (CODs) in LGBTQ people, many clinicians will likely need to expand their cultural expertise. To address some of these issues, this chapter will focus on three cases that highlight some of the pertinent issues.

## Clinical Case 1

Nic is a 35-year-old gay man who was referred to an outpatient mental health clinic after at least four psychiatric hospitalizations that were marked by disorganization, auditory hallucinations, and substance abuse. He was most recently diagnosed with schizophrenia.

Nic grew up in a rural town and was raised by a single mother who suffered from alcoholism. Nic described himself as a "quiet rebel" while growing up in that he avoided criticism but never really trusted his teachers, mother, or classmates, who he felt would be critical if he "came out." After graduating from a local college with good grades, Nic moved to an urban area, where he got a job as an accountant. At night, he began to use "party drugs" and engage in risky sexual activity, as well as group sex with strangers. He often had unprotected receptive anal intercourse, and eventually contracted HIV. His preferred drugs included ecstasy, cocaine, and crystal methamphetamine. After the diagnosis of HIV, Nic reduced his use of party drugs. He did continue to use crystal meth almost daily, which he said helped him focus in addition to improving his sexual experiences. He was able to maintain his job until age 30, when an episode of agitated psychosis led to a hospitalization and a job termination.

In the outpatient psychiatric department, Nic reported auditory hallucinations, mood lability, and occasional suicidal thoughts. He agreed to weekly psychotherapy and medication management. The focus of treatment was to reduce crystal meth use through motivational interviewing and to treat symptoms with antipsychotic medication and mood stabilizers.

Despite months of harm reduction treatment, group therapy, and medication management, Nic would still use crystal meth several times a week. He was frequently non-adherent to medication and would suffer from auditory hallucinations that mainly distracted him from work.

Given his inability to stop drug use and nonadherence to medication, Nic is started on an injectable antipsychotic. After 2 months of treatment, his auditory hallucinations subside, and he is able to maintain regular work despite a previous inability to keep a job. Nic continues to struggle with crystal meth addiction, but his overall level of functioning has increased with injectable medication.

# Discussion

"Crystal meth," or methamphetamine, is considered by many to be a "super cocaine" that not only causes dopamine receptor stimulation but also floods the brain with dopamine. It is a highly addictive drug that can cause psychotic symptoms of hallucinations and paranoia. Crystal meth use has been prevalent among the gay population, especially when associated with unprotected and group sex activities. It helps with confidence, stamina, and physical pleasure. It can be injected, also called "slamming," which can make the experience more intense. The crash that follows can mimic severe depression, even suicidal feelings, with lingering psychosis and physical exhaustion.

Patients like Nic frequently end up at an emergency room, where their psychotic symptoms can be mistaken for schizophrenia or bipolar disorder. It is important to identify the timing of the psychotic symptoms. Did they occur before or after the first use of crystal meth? Do they continue after a period of sobriety? In regards to Nic, his psychotic symptoms developed in the context of cocaine and ecstasy use, as well as the crystal meth, and although the psychotic symptoms have persisted, he has not had a prolonged period of sobriety.

In regard to DSM-5, Nic appears to have had multiple diagnoses: stimulant use disorder (crystal methamphetamine and cocaine) and hallucinogen use disorder (ecstasy), as well as substance-induced psychotic disorder. Although he may eventually be diagnosed with a primary psychotic disorder, his symptoms do not qualify for a diagnosis of schizophrenia or bipolar disorder until his psychosis persists in the absence of the use of a substance known to induce psychosis.

When treating crystal meth addiction with conventional substance abuse interventions, clinicians may become frustrated by recurrent relapses. Patients may seem to be making progress, disappear from treatment, and repeatedly return for additional treatment. Crystal meth is such an addictive drug that harm reduction is sometimes the only workable method of treatment. An important part of the treatment is for the clinician to avoid discouragement, maintain a connection with the patient, and remain aware of such motivational interviewing principles as remaining nonjudgmental and "rolling with resistance." This approach can be especially true for people, like Nic, who have ambivalence toward people in authority and a seemingly intractable addiction to the crystal meth.

Injectable depot antipsychotic medication is sometimes used for people with both psychotic symptoms and ongoing abuse of crystal methamphetamine. The underlying rationale for this strategy is that the antipsychotic medication will still be physiologically available even if the patient is actively relapsing, which might prevent worsening psychosis both during and after the drug use. This approach is not yet supported by evidence, but anecdotally it seems to have merit.

Another unconventional approach to refractory meth amphetamine addiction is to try to curb cravings by offering other stimulants. For example, a tablet of methamphetamine can be offered with the rationale that it may provide enough craving relief to prevent the patient from "slamming" a large amount of crystal meth and going on a 3-day drug bender. If the functionality of the patient increases overall with no additional harm done to the patient, it would be deemed successful care.

Nic is described as using crystal meth for focus and concentration. The case report does not clarify whether he carries an additional diagnosis of attention-deficit/hyperactivity disorder (ADHD) or whether his concentration difficulties are more likely to be secondary to his illicit substance use. Either way, it is clinically important to attend to all of Nic's reported difficulties, including ones that may seem relatively unimportant to the clinician. While more conservative psychiatrists may refuse to prescribe stimulants when working with any patient with a substance abuse history, it can be quite useful to treat a diagnosis of ADHD that may be driving some of the substance abuse.

Clinicians who work with people in the LGBTQ community also need to be aware of their own judgments. In the case of Nic, his clinicians will need to address their own views on sex parties. The clinician's approach should be to promote safety while recognizing patient preference. For example, therapy might include discussion of ways to incorporate safe-sex practices and sobriety into desired sexual activities. A clinician who is judgmental of sexual practices runs the risk of having the patient withhold important information and possibly losing the patient from care altogether.

## Clinical Case 2

Elaine is a 22-year-old woman who presents to outpatient psychiatry for treatment of severe agoraphobia and opioid dependence. She has a history of hospitalizations secondary to suicidal ideation and anxiety attacks.

Elaine was raised as a boy but always knew she was a girl. She grew up in a rural area, where no one in her family or community had experience with Elaine's gender diversity. Her parents were extremely religious and concluded that Elaine was possessed by the devil. By age 12, Elaine was using information from the Internet to argue that she was not mentally ill or possessed but simply transgender. In response, her parents forced her to undergo "reparative therapy" in which a psychologist attempted to convince her she was male.

After a year of reparative therapy and ongoing bullying at school and home for being "sissy," Elaine ran away at age 13. Without resources, she became homeless in a large urban area. She connected with other homeless trans and gay youth, who introduced her to sex work, which allowed her to support herself and to get hold of feminizing hormones, which she obtained from the street.

Elaine's clients were typically older men who used substances during sex. Occasional use of heroin quickly led to heroin dependence, and she spent several years in difficult circumstances marked by physical abuse, panic, and prolonged bouts of agoraphobia that greatly restricted her mobility. She was hospitalized multiple times for suicidality and panic, generally in the context of heroin abuse and conflicts with sexual partners. At age 20, after obtaining steady housing and trans-affirming services, Elaine detoxed from heroin with the help of buprenorphine.

Over the prior year, Elaine reports more stability than she has ever had, but the anxiety attacks persist. She has also become more able to talk about the difficulties of being transgender. Derogatory comments and physical threats occur almost daily, and she believes it is almost impossible for her to get a stable job because of her trans identity. In addition, when she does get a retail job, her frequent panic attacks make it difficult to get to work on time. This leads to continued sex work to pay her bills. The panic and agoraphobia also make it difficult to see her psychiatrist to get buprenorphine. Missed appointments lead to withdrawal which leads her to pursue other opioids.

---

# Discussion

Much of the clinical work with Elaine is similar to that with any other patient who has CODs. It is, however, useful to understand some basics of the transgender experience.

In describing Elaine as "trans," the clinician should recognize that Elaine was identified by her parents as a boy at birth and that she presumably has XY chromosomes (i.e., her "natal gender" was male). The word "trans" is used in contrast to the word "cis," which refers to people whose own gender identity is concordant with that which he or she was raised as a child. In the LGBTQ community, Nic from the first case would be referred to as a cis gay man, while Madison in the upcoming case would be described as a "cis woman" or "cis lesbian." This terminology is not uniformly used but is an effort to avoid "exceptionalizing" the trans experience.

The case report indicates that Elaine describes her childhood behavior as "sissy." While friends and family may view "gender atypical" behavior as completely acceptable, it continues to be the case that "sissy" boys and "tomboy" girls continue to face childhoods marked by teasing and bullying that can be ruthless. As is the case for Elaine, transgender and gender nonconforming (TGNC) individuals often have psychiatric after-effects of early childhood abuse (James et al. 2016). For Elaine, the abuse began at home and intensified after she ran away and became a homeless 13-year-old sex worker.

Children with gender atypical behavior during childhood may never question their own gender identity, and they may later describe their adult sexual orientation as gay, straight, or bisexual (i.e., gender identity and sexual object choice are not inevitably linked). The case report does not actually clarify Elaine's sexual orientation. Lifelong (or "early onset") women of trans experience are generally attracted primarily or only to men, but trans women who are late-onset (i.e., they recognize they are trans as adolescents or adults) are often primarily attracted to cis or trans women. As is true in the larger cis community, trans people may also describe themselves as bisexual. If trying to clarify sexual orientation, it is generally useful to ask about fantasies rather than just focus on behavior. For example, the fact that Elaine only mentions having had sex with men may primarily reflect the realities of sex work rather than her own sexual orientation.

*Transgender* is an umbrella term for a transient or persistent identification that is different from one's natal gender. Pronoun choice is determined by Elaine: she's a she because she identifies as a woman. *Transsexual* refers to an individual who seeks or has undergone a social transition between the genders. This is a social construct and not related to surgery or the use of hormones. This word is not typically used in the transgender community, as the option of surgery and/or hormones is just one facet to the overall gender spectrum and identifying as transgender. LGBTQ also includes a more fluid perspective on both gender identity and sexual orientation. *Queer* and *questioning* people tend to reject simple sexual binaries. When the clinician is uncertain about pronoun usage, definitions, or any other aspect of the LGBTQ world, the clinician can simply ask.

*Gender dysphoria* is the only DSM-5 diagnosis that specifically applies to transgender individuals. It is a controversial term. It can be useful, as when it eases the path for trans people to use insurance for hormones and surgery, and when it provides legal protection for trans people who have experienced discrimination. Furthermore, the term is intended to focus on the dysphoria related to the gender discordance rather than to be a commentary on all transgender people. It can be argued, however, that there are no longer DSM-5 diagnoses for people who are dissatisfied about being gay and that gender dysphoria may be a term that unnecessarily pathologizes people within the trans community.

Elaine spent a year in "reparative therapy," which is a type of treatment that tries to change gender identity or sexual orientation. It is yet to be known the mechanism by which someone develops their sexual orientation or gender identity, but it is well known that reparative therapy is psychologically damaging to individuals and can even lead to suicide (Scasta and Bialer 2013).

Elaine's case report does not clarify her inner experience of being transgender but instead focuses on her behaviors and difficulties. Running away from home at age 13, Elaine became a sex worker, which is a not uncommon way for TGNC youth to support themselves. Transgender people have become widely fetishized, and there is a demand for their services. In addition to the many risks involved in sex work, Elaine also developed an opiate use disorder, which may have been a way for her to control her anxiety and to numb herself during the sex. The heroin may have also been cynically and knowingly offered by an adult: prostitution is illegal, as is sex with 13-year-old children, and one way to increase the likelihood that Elaine would avoid authorities would be to have her dependent on heroin.

At about the same time that she was injecting heroin, Elaine started buying injectable feminizing hormones from street dealers. Without either trans-affirming healthcare or parental consent, many trans teens obtain street hormones. We do not know Elaine's medical history, but HIV and hepatitis are commonly seen in people with her life experience.

Alliance building can be difficult in working with people who have been chronically abused. In addition to the opiate use disorder, she seems to most clearly identify her problems as related to anxiety and agoraphobia. These warrant attention, and she may benefit from medications and psychotherapy that target these disorders. It might also be very useful to listen to her perspectives on being targeted from such a young age, just as it might be useful to try to better understand her suicidal feelings, her relationship issues, and any other CODs, such as posttraumatic stress disorder.

## Clinical Case 3

Madison is a 22-year-old college senior who presented to her university psychiatric clinic for treatment of alcohol abuse and mood swings. Over the prior summer, she had been diagnosed with borderline personality disorder, bipolar disorder, and alcohol use disorder by her hometown psychiatrist. She had been taking lamotrigine for 2 months.

Madison said that she had been fine until a couple of years earlier. Growing up in a fundamentalist religious home, she had not been exposed to alcohol until she went away to college. During her freshman year, she drank the occasional beer, but by sophomore year, she had escalated her alcohol use. By junior year, she was experiencing blackouts, social isolation, and poor grades. She says that she was single but that she had just broken up with a girlfriend. She said that break-up had been "stormy," which led her to feeling desperate. She says that while intoxicated, she occasionally cut her arms, got into screaming fights, and expressed the wish to be dead. Her friends and family were shocked by this behavior, since she had always been quiet and shy. Twice over the summer, her parents had called an ambulance because she seemed suicidal. During that second emergency room visit, in early August, a psychiatrist had diagnosed a bipolar disorder, borderline personality disorder, and alcohol abuse. She had been started on lamotrigine and olanzapine.

Madison told the on-campus psychiatrist in September that her biggest issue was not that she was manic, depressed, suicidal, or drinking too much alcohol. She said the problem was her girlfriend. In particular, she was distraught that her girlfriend no longer spoke to her. She said they were wonderful together except for the fact that they had been forced to keep the relationship a complete secret, which ultimately frustrated the girlfriend and led to the breakup. Madison added that she had told her family that she was a lesbian when she was a freshman but that they had become enraged and threatened to cut her off financially and never speak to her again if she didn't "come to her senses." To address their concerns, Madison never again mentioned anything about dating women. She had dated some local men, but she found these experiences to be a pale reminder of her girlfriend.

While her relationship issues most upset Madison, she did admit to drinking at least half a liter of vodka every day, with blackout and withdrawal tremors. She also described often feeling empty, desperate, impulsive, and angry. She also found herself feeling suicidal, especially while feeling lonely and intoxicated.

The on-campus therapist identified several issues that warranted attention. Alcohol use disorder received individual therapy with a focus on motivational interviewing, a referral to Alcoholics Anonymous (AA), and medication-assisted therapy (she received acamprosate). Since her other symptoms had developed in the context of the alcohol use disorder, he diagnosed her with alcohol-induced depressive disorder and deferred clarifying a personality disorder and a bipolar disorder. He continued the lamotrigine but discontinued the olanzapine after a few weeks. He also referred her for weekly psychotherapy.

Madison was initially ambivalent about the therapy, which had been presented to her as "LGBTQ affirming." She, herself, was not completely sure that she was interested in "being affirmed" as part of a lesbian community—she said she just needed to "stop getting drunk" and not kill herself. Over the next few months, she stopped drinking alcohol, partly because of therapy and the acamprosate, but also because she found a home group and sponsor within AA. She said the home group was an LGBTQ group "but was otherwise totally normal." Mood swings, dysphoria, and angry outbursts persisted but did improve. Madison's suicidality also seemed to dissipate within weeks, though it reappeared when she tried unsuccessfully to date other women. Over the next few months, Madison was surprised to find that she often felt "normal." By March of the next semester, her psychiatrist decided that her mood symptoms had been secondary to the alcohol use and discontinued the lamotrigine. The following summer, Madison elected to stay on campus to continue with her therapy and home group and to work in a college internship. While she had been encouraged by some of her friends to come out to her family, she decided that she would rather just not get into it with them. Six months after the lamotrigine was discontinued, Madison remained euthymic and sober, at which point her psychiatrist discontinued the acamprosate.

# Discussion

The "coming out" process can be stormy, especially if done in an unsupportive environment. Mood lability, impulsivity, angry outbursts, and even suicidal ideation are not uncommon and can lead many psychiatrists to diagnose the patient with a wide variety of diagnoses. Like straight patients, LGBTQ patients can have any DSM-5 diagnosis, but it is useful to remember that many acute symptoms resolve when the patient finds a more affirming environment. Madison is a good example of this.

Alcohol use disorder is common in the LGBTQ population for several reasons. Alcohol can help suppress sexual feelings in people who are trying to avoid sex. For other people, alcohol can also reduce inhibitions enough to have sex. Culturally, many LGBTQ people have learned to socialize around drinking establishments. For an isolated and closeted person, a gay bar may be the only available and safe environment to meet people. LGBTQ people in recovery or harm reduction programs are frequently faced with having to navigate a gay world that can seem to revolve around alcohol. Larger cities have social groups and LGBTQ centers that offer alternatives, but in a small rural town, the local gay bar may be the only place to reliably find other people who are LGBTQ.

Although the coming out process can be difficult, it can also be surprisingly easy—many men and women have worried about coming out only to have their loved ones respond with complete support and often a lack of surprise. However, even if a person's immediate family and friends are supportive, they still might live in a largely homophobic environment depending on their location and cultural surroundings.

While recognizing the difficulties of the coming out process, mental health clinicians still need to look for all treatable diagnoses. In Madison's case, the psychiatrist didn't normalize the drinking, for example, and began treatment with multiple therapies, including psychotherapy, AA, and acamprosate. Similarly, the psychiatrist accepted the possibility that Madison had other underlying psychiatric diagnoses. Although the olanzapine, lamotrigine, and acamprosate were eventually discontinued, they were discontinued sequentially over many months, and only after a significant period of euthymia and abstinence.

# Conclusion

Working with the LGBTQ population in the context of co-occurring disorders can be challenging. Finding sexual orientation and gender-affirming treatments is difficult outside of large cities, and most clinicians receive little to no education in LGBTQ mental health during their professional training. The LGBTQ population is disproportionately affected when it comes to substance use disorders due to several factors. Two of these factors include societal stigma with nonacceptance and the lack of safe spaces to meet other LGBTQ people outside of drinking establishments or gay bars. When treating co-occurring disorders in the LGBTQ population, clinicians need to think about their treatment planning through the lens of gender and sexual orientation diversity. Some of the more common treatment methods might not apply to LGBTQ people, and triggers can be present that are not typical in a straight-cis population. Clinicians will need to be mindful of their patients' particular stressors and life situations.

## KEY POINTS

- Treatment of co-occurring disorders in the LGBTQ community warrants awareness of cultural differences and an individual approach to care.

- Crystal methamphetamine is a powerfully addictive drug that is commonly used by urban gay men as part of a sex party scene.

- Transgender individuals commonly suffer years of trauma that can begin in childhood and have life-long implications.

- LGBTQ individuals going through the coming out process can suffer from a wide range of symptoms that may mimic personality disorders, mood disorders, and anxiety disorders.

- Reparative therapy is damaging and can potentially lead to suicide.

# Questions

1. A transgender male patient who has been taking testosterone by intramuscular means for several years now has developed crystal meth addiction and has been known to inject or "slam" the drug. In your treatment, what should you suggest about testosterone?

    A. Advise him to stop testosterone. It is likely leading to the crystal meth addiction.
    B. Look for other forms of testosterone treatment. Injecting the medication may be a trigger.

C. Continue intramuscular testosterone. There is no need for further assessment when providing trans-affirming care.

D. Consider that he is abusing testosterone in addition to crystal meth.

2. A young cisgender teenager who recently started to explore his sexual feelings discovered that he is attracted to other boys and has tried to keep it a secret from his family and friends because of their strict religious associations. He started using alcohol with his friends and was noticed to drink large amounts and have blackouts. He was taken to the emergency room one night because his parents noticed him recently having mood swings and they discovered he has been telling friends at school he is thinking about suicide. What should be the first steps with this patient?

A. Think about prescribing a mood stabilizer. He may be suffering from bipolar disorder and a medication like lithium could prevent suicide.

B. Refer him to reparative therapy. If a therapist can help him have feelings toward girls, his suicidality will resolve.

C. Arrange a family meeting to clarify the patient's homosexuality.

D. Create a safety plan around suicide and start LGBTQ-affirming care. Allow him to discuss his feelings in an open and nonjudgmental environment.

3. A 35-year-old cisgender gay man comes to an outpatient clinic with crystal meth addiction. He uses crystal meth when he is sexually active, and this causes him to have intense hallucinations and paranoia. He recently lost his job and is facing homelessness due to the addiction. Which is the best possible treatment available to this patient?

A. Crystal Meth Anonymous.

B. Abstinence program.

C. Antipsychotic medication.

D. Stimulants.

E. Motivational interviewing.

F. Group therapy.

G. Selective serotonin reuptake inhibitors.

H. All of the above.

# References

James SE, Herman JL, Rankin S, et al: Executive Summary of the Report of the 2015 U.S. Transgender Survey. Washington, DC, National Center for Transgender Equality, 2016

Scasta D, Bialer P: Position statement on issues related to homosexuality. American Psychiatric Association, 2013

# 18

# INCARCERATION

### *Lauren Stossel, M.D.*

Mental health efforts with incarcerated patients who have substance use disorders (SUDs) are complicated by the reality that both the patient and the clinician are working within an institutional setting that complicates the normal clinician–patient relationship. Incarcerated patients have limited mobility and access to care, of course, while clinicians are faced with a limited medication formulary and regulations that restrict treatments (Ford 2015; Friedmann et al. 2012; Gray et al. 2014). Clinicians must also come to terms with "dual loyalties," in that they have obligations both to their patient and to the correctional staff, which can—at times—lead to inevitable conflict (Pont et al. 2012).

Work within a correctional setting also requires expanding a knowledge base beyond that of most mental health practitioners. For example, the clinician will learn about jails, which are short-term facilities that house people who have been newly arrested, sentenced to less than a year, or are awaiting disposition of their criminal cases (Cornelius 2012; Ford 2015). Sixty percent of jail inmates have not been convicted of a crime and are awaiting action on their criminal cases; they do not have a discharge date (Ford 2015; Minton and Zeng 2015). Jails differ from state and federal prisons, which are longer-term facilities that house sentenced inmates. In addition to learning necessary details about correctional institutions, the clinician who treats incarcerated patients will also need to develop a working relationship with members of the criminal justice system who they might never otherwise meet.

It is important that incarcerated patients have access to psychiatric treatment for co-occurring disorders (CODs). For example, almost half of incarcerated patients have symptoms that meet criteria for both a SUD and a primary mental disorder (James and Glaze 2006). Of those with a mental disorder, 75% also have a SUD (James and Glaze 2006). Over a third of incarcerated patients were using substances at the time of their alleged crime (James and Glaze 2006). Clinicians who work with this population need to be prepared for the reality that complex clinical presentations are routine (see Figure 18–1 later in this chapter).

In addition to the many challenges, the criminal justice system may also provide people with CODs an important opportunity for treatment. Their diagnoses may be recognized for the first time, and legal incentives may motivate the patient to begin recovery (Center for Substance Abuse Treatment 2005; Ford 2015). For others, arrest and incarceration may be a part of a long-standing cycle of substance use and illegal behavior. Clinicians may need to creatively develop broad, intensive, and integrated treatment approaches to help with ingrained patterns of maladaptive coping skills and criminal values that further complicate the CODs (Center for Substance Abuse Treatment 2005).

In the following case, we describe a young man with schizophrenia and multiple SUDs who works his way through a variety of institutional settings. In the discussion, we focus on treatments and negotiations that are typical within the justice system—and unusual outside of that system. Although the case is specific to this young man, the underlying principles can be considered when working with any incarcerated patient.

---

## Clinical Case

Frank is a 35-year-old single man, domiciled in supportive housing and tenuously employed as a mover for a furniture company. He has an unclear psychiatric history and no readily available collateral information. He is charged with felony possession of a narcotic. Unable to make bail, he is incarcerated in a city jail to await trial.

During his initial psychiatric screen, his speech is loud and pressured and he exhibits significant psychomotor agitation.

He describes his mood as "anxious" and endorses paranoid delusions of government surveillance and auditory hallucinations of several threatening male voices. He denies suicidal and homicidal ideation. He admits to daily alcohol use of "a pint or two." He also uses heroin regularly. For both heroin and alcohol, he uses whatever he "can get and pay for." He last used heroin about 4 hours prior to incarceration but denies alcohol use the day of his arrest. His urine toxicology is positive for opiates. His blood alcohol level at the time of initial booking is 0.

A few hours into his evaluation, Frank becomes agitated and gets into a verbal altercation with another inmate. On initial physical examination, he is noted to be diaphoretic, tremulous, and mildly hypertensive and tachycardic. While perhaps related to the fight with the other inmate, the symptoms and his negative alcohol level lead to a presumptive diagnosis of alcohol withdrawal. Frank accepts chlordiazepoxide for treatment of presumptive alcohol withdrawal. Later that same day, he also exhibits diarrhea, nausea, and muscle cramping, which are symptoms of opiate withdrawal. Frank is transferred to a detoxification unit to help him get safely off both alcohol and heroin. He is not offered methadone maintenance because he has been charged with a felony. During the detox, Frank undergoes an extended evaluation to monitor withdrawal and suicidality and to try to determine his psychiatric baseline and the extent to which his symptoms are attributable to substance use. Review of jail records reveals Frank has two prior incarcerations for misdemeanor charges. He also describes a history of childhood physical abuse with resultant posttraumatic stress disorder (PTSD), intermittent homelessness, chronic schizophrenia, at least one prior suicide attempt, and marijuana, opiate, and alcohol use disorders. After 1 week, he is transferred to the general jail population.

Frank continues to suffer from psychotic symptoms during the weeks after he is detoxified from the alcohol and heroin. Because of the persistence of psychosis, he is transferred to a "mental observation" housing unit for inmates with serious mental illness (SMI). Frank's psychotic symptoms persist but do improve over the next few weeks with consistent medication adherence, sobriety, and the structured setting.

Over the ensuing months, however, Frank gets into repeated arguments with corrections officers and other inmates. It is also noted that he repeatedly misses medication doses and has repeatedly tested positive for contraband substances (mostly opioids). After several months in jail, Frank decides to stop his medications because they are "poison." In the absence of anti-psychotic medication, Frank stops bathing, refuses meals, and will not leave his cell for treatment groups. He is transferred to a nearby psychiatric hospital for stabilization.

Following stabilization on the inpatient unit, Frank returns to jail. Given his earlier clinical improvement, Frank's city-appointed defense attorney proposes drug treatment court enrollment, and the district attorney accepts. Frank meets eligibility criteria because of his opiate use and nonviolent drug-related offense. Frank accepts a guilty plea and is released from jail. The drug court follows Frank for 18 months, during which time he attends monthly hearings in front of the presiding judge. He also begins methadone maintenance treatment and adheres to a treatment and monitoring protocol that includes random and scheduled drug testing and mandatory attendance at a drug treatment program. Frank completes the program and his conviction is overturned and removed from his record.

# Discussion

Because Frank has been charged but not convicted of a crime, he is incarcerated in a jail setting. Stress within jails is related to incarceration, of course, but also to uncertainty among inmates. When will they be released? Will they be convicted? Even if not convicted, the incarcerated patient can lose a hard-earned job or custody of a child. Turnover rates are high within jails, and inmates are often shuffled between housing units (Center for Substance Abuse Treatment 2005; Ford 2015). Frequent movement contributes to a high-anxiety atmosphere, especially for people with a baseline mental illness (Center for Substance Abuse Treatment 2005; Ford 2015). The mentally ill are also disproportionately exposed to various types of trauma in jail settings (Gosein et al. 2016).

In contrast to jails, state and federal prisons hold offenders who are sentenced to serve more than 1 year. Because of the longer period of incarceration and known, definite release date, prisons provide more stability (Center for Substance Abuse Treatment 2005). They also tend to provide greater opportunity for mental health assessment, diagnosis, and treatment (Center for Substance Abuse Treatment 2005). In-prison drug abuse treatment, particularly when followed by community-based continuing care treatment, has been credited with reducing short-term recidivism and relapse rates among offenders who are involved with drugs (Beck and Maruschak 2001; Center for Substance Abuse Treatment 2005).

## DIAGNOSTIC EVALUATION

Frank presents with psychotic symptoms in the context of alcohol and heroin use disorders. Pending collateral history and clinical progress, the differential diagnosis includes substance-induced psychotic disorder, primary psychotic disorder, and mood disorder with psychotic features, along with the SUDs. To clarify the diagnosis, it is important to monitor Frank's psychotic symptoms after his intoxication clears. Within the jail, this psychiatric screening is an initial step before referral to further mental health services (Ford 2015). Frank also warrants close observation in the immediate aftermath of his incarceration, since he is at increased risk for suicide, particularly due to his substance use history (European Monitoring Center for Drugs and Drug Addiction 2006; U.S. Department of Justice 2010).

Frank's diagnostic evaluation is facilitated by the existence of records from his previous incarcerations. In the absence of these, his mental health history might have been more difficult to obtain, especially since collateral information from family and community providers tends to become less available after an arrest (Ford 2015). One legal issue pertinent to treatment of the incarcerated patient is the fact that community treatment programs can share records with corrections facilities without patient consent (Ford 2015; U.S. Department of Health and Human Services 2002). This provision within the Health Insurance Portability and Accountability Act (HIPAA) is an effort to ensure continuity of care after incarcerated patients are abruptly removed from their community treatment by their arrest (Ford 2015; U.S. Department of Health and Human Services 2002). This HIPAA exception may reduce what would otherwise increase the likelihood of symptom recurrence (Gray et al. 2014). Many community treatment programs are unaware of this HIPAA exception and therefore may fail to provide helpful documentation. For different reasons, family members of incarcerated patients may be difficult to locate and/or may be hesitant to be entirely forthcoming when discussing their loved ones' psychiatric history (Gray et al. 2014).

Records are particularly important because actual rates of mental disorders in incarcerated populations are likely to be higher than self-reported rates (Center for Substance Abuse Treatment 2005). There is significant stigma associated with mental disorders within the prison and jail culture, and inmates may hide symptoms or a psychiatric history to avoid being victimized by peers (Center for Substance Abuse Treatment 2005; Chaiken et al. 2005; Ford 2015). Substance abuse does not carry the same degree of stigma in correctional facilities as it does in the community. Because one disorder can mask or imitate the other, accurate diagnosis of co-occurring mental illness in inmates with SUDs requires skilled screening and assessment (Center for Substance Abuse Treatment 2005). Additionally, providers in a correctional setting must be mindful of inmates who may exaggerate symptoms in order to obtain advantages, such as less restrictive housing (Chaiken et al. 2005; Ford 2015).

Frank's diagnosis of schizophrenia would classify him as a patient with serious mental illness (SMI). SMI is generally defined in correctional settings as a mental or behavioral disorder that results in serious functional impairment, such as schizophrenia, major depressive disorder, and bipolar disorder (American Psychiatric Association 2000). Frank's primary psychotic disorder and substance use disorders are additive and cyclical in their effects on his functional status. His psychotic symptoms impair his executive functioning and increase his anxiety, which he may self-medicate with substances. In turn, his substance use worsens his psychotic symptoms and further compromises his insight and judgment, which leads to discontinuation of antipsychotic medications.

Frank's history of homelessness, physical abuse, and interpersonal conflicts are not uncommon in jails and prisons (James and Glaze 2006). In two ways, Frank's experience is atypical. First, Frank's incarceration is shortened by his participation in drug court. In contrast, recent evidence indicates that people with SMI typically remained incarcerated nearly twice as long as other inmates (Justice Center 2012). In addition, Frank receives treatment for his psychosis during his incarceration. Typically, psychiatric treatment is more the exception than the rule within the U.S. correctional system. One recent study found that people with SMI who are in jail have a one in six chance of receiving psychiatric treatment, while those who are in state prison have a one in three chance of getting treatment for their SMI (James and Glaze 2006).

## WITHDRAWAL

During his initial evaluation phase, Frank experiences withdrawal symptoms related to alcohol and opiate dependence. Withdrawal symptoms often begin before arrestees like Frank have been formally charged with a crime (which may take up to 72 hours), much less convicted. The implicit threat of withdrawal after detention may lead arrestees into providing information they might not otherwise volunteer (Center for Substance Abuse Treatment 2005). Although guidelines exist, detoxification and withdrawal services are often unavailable. Only 28% of jail administrators reported that their jails provided alcohol or drug detoxification services. While standards for jails and prisons in regard to management of withdrawal have been established by the NCCHC, only 8% of U.S. jails have obtained accreditation. After weighting of jail size estimates, Fiscella et al. (2004) estimated that 63% of all U.S. arrestees were detained in facilities which reported never detoxifying inmates. A 2004 report from the Bureau of Justice Statistics reported that less than 1% of inmates who admitted abusing drugs or alcohol at the time of arrest reported receiving detoxification in jail (James 2004).

## CRIMINAL DIVERSION PROGRAMS

Because of his nonviolent, drug-related charge and SUD, Frank was eligible to participate in a drug treatment court. Eligible inmates can be diverted to drug courts when their attorney presents this as an alternative to incarceration to the district attorney. Enrollment in drug court involves taking a guilty plea, participating in treatment, and appearing monthly for drug testing and hearing before a judge for an average of 18 months. If, like Frank, inmates adhere with the program guidelines until completion, the conviction is overturned and comes off the individual's record. Those who don't comply are remanded to jail where they may serve a reduced or full sentence (Figure 18–1).

In the United States, diversion programs have become increasingly popular as a means of diverting nonviolent offenders away from jails and prisons into more treatment-oriented settings (Ford 2015; Matusow et al. 2013). Diversion programs typically fall into two categories: prebooking and postbooking (Ford 2015). *Prebooking diversion* programs are geared toward reducing the number of arrests. One successful example of this is Crisis Intervention Training (CIT), in which police officers are trained to recognize signs and symptoms of mental illness in the field, de-escalate mentally ill individuals in crisis, and facilitate referral to treatment services (Council of State Governments 2002; Watson et al. 2010). *Postbooking diversion* programs involve alternatives to incarceration, such as drug courts and mental health courts (Ford 2015).

The National Drug Court Institute (NDCI) estimates that in 2009, more than 116,000 criminal offenders were served by a drug court program (Huddleston and Marlowe 2011). Aggregated data suggest that drug and mental health courts reduce illicit drug use and recidivism and improve adherence to treatment (Carey et al. 2008; Ford 2015; Matusow et al. 2013; Steadman et al. 2011).

## FOLLOW-UP

While Frank's future is uncertain, he is at risk for relapse and overdose upon reentry into the community. Approximately one-third of inmates re-

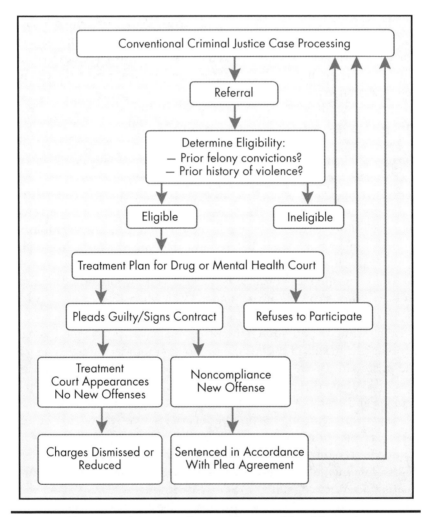

FIGURE 18–1.    **Pathway to drug and mental health court.**

sume substance abuse within the first 2 months of their release, and 95% of those incarcerated for drug crimes return to drug use within 3 years of their release (Marlowe 2003; Matusow et al. 2013). Opioid overdose risk increases sevenfold during the first 2 weeks following release from the incarceration (Matusow et al. 2013; Sporer and Kral 2007). In a study of mortality rates in more than 76,000 individuals released from prisons in Washington State, the overdose rate of recently released inmates (2 weeks) was nearly 13 times that of the general population (Binswanger et al. 2013). Various treatment modalities may mitigate the risks over relapse and overdose.

# Treatment

## INCARCERATION SETTING

The jail setting creates unique challenges associated with treatment in addition to the challenges particular to diagnostic evaluation. These include availability of and adherence to medication and therapy, as well as continuity with community treatment (Center for Substance Abuse Treatment 2005; Ford 2015).

Appropriate treatment services differ based on setting and where the offender is in the criminal justice pathway. In the pretrial setting, the question of an individual's guilt or innocence has not been legally determined. Treatment professionals need to bear in mind the presumption of innocence that exists during the pretrial period. Defendants' due process rights may affect what they are willing to agree to and the type of information that they are willing to disclose. Defendants should not be coerced into waiving due process rights, although a court may order substance abuse treatment as a condition of pretrial release (Center for Substance Abuse Treatment 2005).

## TREATMENT OPTIONS IN JAIL

In a jail setting, treatment options are relatively limited. Brief treatment (less than 30 days) usually focuses on supplying information and making referrals, but can include motivational interviewing. Short-term programs (1–3 months) work on communication, problem-solving, relapse prevention skills, anger management techniques, and participation in self-help groups. It is important that these short-term treatment programs also include linkage to community resources.

One important facet of substance use treatment in the jail setting is *detoxification*. While, as discussed earlier, these services are rare, they are not impossible to implement. For example, the Key Extended Entry Program (KEEP) at Rikers Island in New York City has been continuously operating since 1987. It has provided, on average, 18,000 detoxifications per year and referred thousands to community-based treatment upon release (Mitchell et al. 2009).

## TREATMENT OPTIONS IN PRISON

Because of the comparative stability of the prison population, treatment options of differing intensities can be made available. These include comprehensive assessment; treatment planning; placement; group, individual, family, and specialty group counseling; self-help groups; educational and vocational training; and planning for transition to the community. Therapeutic communities (TCs) are among the most successful in-prison treatment programs. They are highly structured, hierarchical, and intense interventions lasting a minimum of 6 months. TC participants live together, often separate from the general prison population, and take responsibility for their recovery process. In-prison drug abuse treatment, particularly when followed by community-based continuing care treatment, has been credited with reducing short-term recidivism and relapse rates among offenders who are involved with drugs (Center for Substance Abuse Treatment 2005; Office of National Drug Control Policy 1999).

For inmates with CODs like Frank, there has been rapid growth in corrections-based co-occurring programs. One study compared a modified therapeutic community (MTC) program for dually diagnosed prison inmates with treatment as usual and with a mental health group. The MTC group was found to have fewer new arrests, less use of illicit drugs, and better compliance with treatment regimens (S. Sacks, J. Peters, H. Wexler, et al.: "Modified Therapeutic Community for MICA Offenders: Description and Interim Findings," unpublished manuscript, 2001). For inmates with psychotic disorders, like Frank, key treatment components include education in drug refusal skills, identification of strategies to fight boredom, building of supportive social networks, and medication adherence (Center for Substance Abuse Treatment 2005).

Several features distinguish the substance abuse programs that specifically treat inmates with CODs. For example, staff from three services (i.e., mental health, substance abuse, and criminal justice) are located in the same program unit and share in decision making. The CODs are treated as "primary," and the treatment is integrated so that both disorders are treated simultaneously. Treatment is generally then adapted to levels of symptom severity, functioning, and commitment to treatment (Center for Substance Abuse Treatment 2005).

Treatment approaches that are commonly used in substance abuse settings (e.g., TCs, cognitive–behavioral treatments, relapse prevention, peer and alumni support groups) can be adapted to suit the needs of dually diagnosed inmates. Common modifications include smaller staff caseloads; shorter, simplified meetings; special attention to criminal thinking; education about medication; and minimizing confrontation (Edens et al. 1997; Peters and Hills 1997). Treatment is provided in graduated stages, using a highly structured psychoeducational approach. Early phases of treatment focus on orientation, assessment, development of treatment plans, and engagement and persuasion activities. Didactic approaches are particularly useful early on to help offenders understand the nature of their mental and substance use disorders. Secondary phases focus more on "active treatment," such as development of coping and life skills, lifestyle change, and cognitive-behavioral interventions. Later phases include relapse prevention, peer mentor activities, vocational training, reentry planning, and linkage with community support and treatment (Center for Substance Abuse Treatment 2005).

## MEDICATION TREATMENT

Medication is an important part of treatment for many dually diagnosed inmates. Patients may have trouble distinguishing between "good" and "bad" drugs, particularly at the beginning of treatment. The distinction is made more difficult by the fact that the "good" medications are more expensive and more difficult to obtain than illicit drugs (Center for Substance Abuse Treatment 2005). An important challenge is the tendency within the substance abuse treatment field to discourage the use of psychotropic medications (Matusow et al. 2013). Programs in criminal justice settings may have outdated formularies, and inmates may not be able to receive necessary medication while incarcerated (Ford 2015). It often takes over a month to be seen by a psychiatrist and receive a prescription for medication, and inmates may not be able to get a sufficient supply upon discharge. Inmates with brief incarcerations may not be followed long enough for certain medications, such as antidepressants, to become effective, and they may not be able to afford medication after release. On the other hand, some inmates may malinger in order to receive medications with "street value," such as benzodiazepines, sedating antidepressants, and some antipsychotics, although many sedating medications are typically unavailable within jails and prisons (Center for Substance Abuse Treatment 2005).

Opioid-assisted treatment (OAT) provides significant benefits but is generally unavailable to the incarcerated population in the United States. The World Health Organization recommends opioid agonist therapy in prisons to reduce risk of HIV transmission and fatal overdose upon release (World Health Organization 2004). There is also evidence that OAT reduces postrelease criminal recidivism and increases the likelihood of postrelease entry into a treatment community (Mitchell et al. 2009).

## REENTRY PLANNING

The last phase of treatment involves helping inmates with CODs with community reentry. In addition to mental health and substance use treatment, planning is required to address concerns related to housing, job skills/placement, and medical needs (Ford 2015). Case management services facilitate access to a broad range of mental health and substance abuse services, and research indicates that they reduce hospitalizations and improve functional status (Mueser et al. 1997).

Recovery and stabilization for dually diagnosed offenders often occurs over several years and multiple treatment episodes. Treatment programs should provide linkage with community treatment and develop detailed aftercare plans to ensure continuity of services and continued access to psychotropic medications. Individuals should be monitored carefully during transition periods, when stress levels are high and there is increased risk for recurrence of symptoms, substance abuse relapse, and criminal recidivism (Center for Substance Abuse Treatment 2005).

Inmates with CODs have particular difficulties finding aftercare programs because of the stigma associated with the combined problems of dual diagnosis and a criminal record (Center for Substance Abuse Treatment 2005). Additionally, many traditional community mental health interventions lack the specialized treatment to address the complex problems that tend to develop in this population (Broner et al. 2002). Community supervision of offenders with CODs requires specialized strategies, including use of supportive rather than confrontational approaches, positive reinforcement for small successes, different expectations regarding response to supervision, flexible responses to infractions, highly structured activities, ongoing monitoring, recruitment of social supports where appropriate, and close coordination between the community supervision/ probation officer and the clinician (Center for Substance Abuse Treatment 2005; Peters and Hills 1997).

# Conclusion

Incarcerated patients with co-occurring mental illness and SUDs are at high risk for morbidity and mortality, have unique diagnostic and treatment needs, and pose unique challenges. In correctional settings, availability of treatment and regulations related to security, policy, and legislation restrict health professionals' ability to provide mental health and substance abuse care as they would in the community. However, for many people with psychiatric disorders and SUDs, contact with the criminal justice system affords them an introduction to treatment. These individuals may be able to take advantage of alternatives to incarceration, which increasingly provide offenders with opportunities to recovery.

# KEY POINTS

- Comorbid mental illness and substance use are extremely common among incarcerated patients. Approximately half of all prisoners in the United States have both a substance abuse problem and a mental illness, and nearly three quarters of incarcerated patients with substance abuse problems are mentally ill.

- In correctional settings, availability of treatment and regulations related to security, policy, and legislation restrict health professionals' ability to provide mental health and substance abuse care as they would in the community.

- Drug courts, mental health courts, and alternatives to incarceration are important options for inmates with co-occurring substance abuse and mental illness. These systems provide therapeutic options for inmates who do not pose a high risk to the community.

- Opiate use disorder is common, and while opioid-assisted treatment is highly effective at preventing relapse and overdose, it is underutilized in prison and jail settings.

# Questions

1. According to the Bureau of Justice Statistics, what percentage of incarcerated individuals with mental illness reported being under the influence of a substance at the time of their offense?

   A. >25%.
   B. >33%.
   C. >50%.
   D. 0%.

2. Which of the following is a difference between a prison and a jail?

   A. Average duration of incarceration.
   B. There are no differences between the two.
   C. Prisons hold more dangerous criminals.
   D. Treatment is more challenging in prisons because inmates do not have a known discharge date.

3.   Which of following is *true* about diversion programs?

A.  Most drug and mental health courts do not offer treatment with agonist medications.

B.  Drug and mental health courts do not reduce illicit drug use and recidivism and fail to improve adherence to treatment.

C.  Most communities have failed to keep diversion programs in operation without federal funding.

D.  Inmates cannot be diverted for mental illness prior to arraignment.

# References

American Psychiatric Association: Psychiatric Services in Jails and prisons, 2nd Edition. Washington, DC, American Psychiatric Association, 2000

Beck AJ, Maruschak LM: Mental Health Treatment in State Prisons, 2000. Washington, DC, Bureau of Justice Statistics, 2001

Binswanger IA, Blatchford PJ, Mueller SR, Stern MF: Mortality after prison release: opioid overdose and other causes of death, risk factors, and time trends from 1999 to 2009. Ann Intern Med 159(9):592–600, 2013 24189594

Broner N, Borum R, Gawley K, et al: A review of screening instruments for co-occurring mental illness and substance use in criminal justice programs, in Serving Mentally Ill Offenders: Challenges and Opportunities for Mental Health Professionals. Edited by Landsberg G, Rock M, Berg L. New York, Springer, 2002, pp 289–337

Carey SM, Finigan MW, Pukstas K: Exploring the key components of drug courts: a comparative study of 18 adult drug courts on practices, outcomes, and costs. NPC Research, March 2008. Available at: https://www.ncjrs.gov/pdffiles1/nij/grants/223853.pdf. Accessed February 7, 2017.

Center for Substance Abuse Treatment: Substance Abuse Treatment for Adults in the Criminal Justice System. Treatment Improvement Protocol (TIP) Series 44 (HHS Publ No SMA-13–4056). Rockville, MD, Substance Abuse and Mental Health Services Administration, 2005

Chaiken SB, Thompson CR, Shoemakers WE: Mental health interventions in correctional settings, in Handbook of Correctional Mental Health. Edited by Scott CL, Gerbasi JB. Washington, DC, American Psychiatric Publishing, 2005, pp 109–131

Cornelius GF: Jails, pre-trial detention, and short term confinement, in The Oxford Handbook of Sentencing and Corrections. Edited by Petersilia J, Reitz KR. New York, Oxford University Press, 2012, pp 389–415

Council of State Governments: Criminal justice/mental health consensus project. June 2002. Available at: https://www.ncjrs.gov/pdffiles1/nij/grants/197103.pdf. Accessed February 7, 2017.

Edens JF, Peters RH, Hills HA: Treating prison inmates with co-occurring disorders: an integrative review of existing programs. Behav Sci Law 15(4):439–457, 1997 9433747

European Monitoring Center for Drugs and Drug Addiction: Clinical management of drug dependence in the adult prison setting: including psychosocial treatment as a core part. Department of Health, November 2006. Available at: file:///C:/Users/marti/Downloads/UK21_management%20in%20prison%20setting.pdf. Accessed February 7, 2017.

Fiscella K, Pless N, Meldrum S, Fiscella P: Alcohol and opiate withdrawal in US jails. Am J Public Health 94(9):1522–1524, 2004 15333308

Ford E: First-episode psychosis in the criminal justice system: identifying a critical intercept for early intervention. Harv Rev Psychiatry 23(3):167–175, 2015 25943312

Friedmann PD, Hoskinson R, Gordon M, et al; MAT Working Group of CJ-DATS: Medication-assisted treatment in criminal justice agencies affiliated with the criminal justice-drug abuse treatment studies (CJ-DATS): availability, barriers, and intentions. Subst Abus 33(1):9–18, 2012 22263709

Gosein VJ, Stiffler JD, Frascoia A, Ford EB: Life Stressors and Posttraumatic Stress Disorder in a Seriously Mentally Ill Jail Population. J Forensic Sci 61(1):116–121, 2016 26280105

Gray SM, Racine CW, Smith CW, Ford EB: Jail hospitalization of prearraignment patient arrestees with mental illness. J Am Acad Psychiatry Law 42(1):75–80, 2014 24618522

Huddleston C, Marlowe D: Painting the current picture: a national report card on drug courts and other problem-solving court programs in the United States. National Drug Court Institute, July 2011. Available at: http://www.ndci.org/sites/default/files/nadcp/PCP%20Report%20FINAL.PDF. Accessed February 7, 2017.

James DJ: Profile of jail inmates, 2002. Bureau of Justice Statistics, 2004. Available at: http://www.bjs.gov/content/pub/pdf/pji02.pdf. Accessed February 7, 2017.

James DJ, Glaze LE: Mental health problems of prison and jail inmates. Bureau of Justice Statistics, 2006. Available at: http://www.bjs.gov/content/pub/pdf/mhppji.pdf. Accessed February 7, 2017.

Justice Center: Improving Outcomes for People with Mental Illnesses Involved with New York City's Criminal Court and Correction Systems. December 2012. Available at: https://csgjusticecenter.org/wp-content/uploads/2013/05/CTBNYC-Court-Jail_7-cc.pdf. Accessed February 7, 2017.

Marlowe DB: Integrating substance abuse treatment and criminal justice supervision. Sci Pract Perspect 2(1):4–14, 2003 18552716

Matusow H, Dickman SL, Rich JD, et al: Medication assisted treatment in US drug courts: results from a nationwide survey of availability, barriers and attitudes. J Subst Abuse Treat 44(5):473–480, 2013 23217610

Minton TD, Zeng Z: Jail inmates at midyear 2014—statistical tables. U.S. Department of Justice, June 2015. Available at: https://www.bjs.gov/content/pub/pdf/jim14.pdf. Accessed February 7, 2017.

Mitchell SG, Kelly SM, Brown BS, et al: Incarceration and opioid withdrawal: the experiences of methadone patients and out-of-treatment heroin users. J Psychoactive Drugs 41(2):145–152, 2009 19705676

Mueser KT, Drake RE, Miles KM: The course and treatment of substance use disorder in persons with severe mental illness, in Treatment of Drug-Dependent Individuals With Comorbid Mental Disorders. NIDA Research Monograph 172 (NIH Publ No 97- 4172). Edited by Onken LS, Blaine JD, Genser S, et al. Rockville, MD, National Institute on Drug Abuse, 1997, pp 86–109

Office of National Drug Control Policy: Therapeutic Communities in Correctional Settings: The Prison Based TC Standards Development Project—Final Report of Phase II. Washington, DC, Office of National Drug Control Policy, 1999

Peters RH, Hills HA: Intervention Strategies for Offenders With Co-Occurring Disorders: What Works? Delmar, NY, National GAINS Center, 1997

Pont J, Stöver H, Wolff H: Dual loyalty in prison health care. Am J Public Health 102(3):475–480, 2012 22390510

Sporer KA, Kral AH: Prescription naloxone: a novel approach to heroin overdose prevention. Ann Emerg Med 49(2):172–177, 2007 17141138

Steadman HJ, Redlich A, Callahan L, et al: Effect of mental health courts on arrests and jail days: a multisite study. Arch Gen Psychiatry 68(2):167–172, 2011 20921111

U.S. Department of Health and Human Services: Corrections, Law Enforcement, and the Courts Health Insurance Portability and Accountability Act of 1996 (HIPAA): 164.512(k)(5) uses and disclosures for correctional institutions and other law enforcement custodial situations. August 14, 2002. Available at: http://www.nga.org/files/live/sites/NGA/files/pdf/FACTSHIPAACORRECT.pdf. Accessed February 7, 2017.

U.S. Department of Justice: National study of jail suicide: 20 years later. April 2010. Available at: http://static.nicic.gov/Library/024308.pdf. Accessed February 7, 2017.

Watson AC, Ottati VC, Morabito M, et al: Outcomes of police contacts with persons with mental illness: the impact of CIT. Adm Policy Ment Health 37(4):302–317, 2010 19705277

World Health Organization: Policy brief: reduction of HIV transmission in prisons. 2004. Available at: http://www.emro.who.int/aiecf/web34.pdf. Accessed February 8, 2017.

# APPENDIX

# ANSWER GUIDE

## Chapter 1

1. Which of the following is an example of the patient's chief complaint?

   A. "My parents are annoying."
   B. 36-year-old man with alcohol use disorder and a history of bipolar disorder.
   C. Recurrent trials of antidepressants and mood stabilizers have failed.
   D. Patient appears sullen, irritable, and with a mild intention tremor.

   **The correct response is option A: "My parents are annoying."**

   The chief complaint is the patient's primary psychiatric concern and is generally written with quotation marks. Even a tangential response can be a window into the patient's mind-set and is therefore helpful to the overall psychiatric evaluation. The chief complaint is specifically not intended to be a brief overall summary, history of treatments, or clinical description.

2. Which of the following components of a psychiatric interview focuses on a cross-sectional assessment of the patient?

    A. History of present illness (HPI).
    B. Mental status exam (MSE).
    C. Assessment.
    D. Treatment plan.

**The correct response is option B: Mental status exam (MSE).**

The MSE is intended to be a cross-sectional perspective on the patient. As such, it is akin to a physical exam. The HPI, assessment, and treatment plan are not cross-sectional. Interestingly, the MSE includes assessments of insight and judgment. Although the clinician can try to assess these cross-sectionally by asking, for example, what patients would do if they were to find a stamped envelope on the sidewalk, it is probably best to look at these more longitudinally. For example, if a patient with a long history of impulsive and thoughtless behavior is able to say that he or she would mail a stamped envelope, their insight and judgment would still be considered "poor."

3.  In the initial assesment of a patient for potentially co-occurring disorders, which one of the following is most crucial to clarify?

    A. The single diagnosis that is causing the most difficulty.
    B. All pertinent psychiatric diagnoses.
    C. Sociopathy and illegal acts that might jeopardize treatment success.
    D. The family's primary concerns.

**The correct response is option B: All pertinent psychiatric diagnoses.**

Central to the initial psychiatric assessment is the recognition of all pertinent psychiatric diagnoses. A core feature of the present volume is the reality that treatment of co-occurring disorders often fails because focus is directed at only one diagnosis. The other issues are also important and should be investigated, but the core issue is making all pertinent diagnoses.

# Chapter 2

1.  What is a core reason to use the Four Quadrant Model of Care for Co-occurring Disorders?

    A. It provides recommendations for psychiatric treatment alone.
    B. It helps clinicians select the appropriate level of care.
    C. It helps determine the stage of change of a patient.
    D. It helps guide medication management.

**The correct response is option B: It helps clinicians select the appropriate level of care.**

The Four Quadrant Model of Care is used to determine the appropriateness of the treatment setting and level of care based on the severity of the substance use disorder (SUD) and psychiatric disorders.

2. What is the value of determining a patient's readiness for change?

    A. It can replace a comprehensive psychiatric evaluation.
    B. It is essential in determining the types of interventions to implement.
    C. It can help the abstinent patient alone maintain abstinence.
    D. It is rarely valuable, as patients with SUDs seldom want to change.

**The correct response is option B: It is essential in determining the types of interventions to implement.**

The determination of a patient's readiness for change is done to identify which stage of change the person is in (precontemplation, contemplation, preparing for action, action, or maintenance) and is important for developing a treatment plan and determining the types of interventions to implement.

3. The 12-step assessment process for co-occurring disorders

    A. Does not include a determination of readiness for change.
    B. Is multidimensional but does not take into account DSM-5.
    C. Is necessary to develop a comprehensive treatment plan.
    D. Includes establishing the diagnoses but not their severity.

**The correct response is option C: Is necessary to develop a comprehensive treatment plan.**

The 12-step assessment process is multidimensional and includes a determination of readiness for change and a determination of

DSM-5 diagnoses and severities. This process is necessary to develop a comprehensive treatment plan.

# Chapter 3

1. Which medication combination has been shown to benefit patients with co-occurring major depressive disorder and alcohol use disorder?

> A. Sertraline and acamprosate.
> B. Desipramine and disulfiram.
> C. Venlafaxine and naltrexone.
> D. Sertraline and naltrexone.

**The correct response is option D: Sertraline and naltrexone.**

Although all of these combinations may benefit patients with major depressive disorder and alcohol use disorder, there is the strongest evidence for sertraline and naltrexone. This medication combination demonstrated improved drinking outcomes, as well as a trend toward significance in improved mood outcomes, in comparison to placebo and to either agent alone.

2. Which psychotherapeutic approach has shown efficacy in three trials of treatment for co-occurring bipolar disorder and SUDs?

> A. Motivational interviewing (MI).
> B. Twelve-step facilitation.
> C. Group drug counseling.
> D. Integrated group therapy (IGT).

**The correct response is option D: Integrated group therapy (IGT).**

A variant of CBT called *integrated group therapy* has demonstrated particular efficacy in the treatment of patients with co-occurring bipolar and substance use disorders. IGT is a 12-session group therapy that strongly emphasizes the interconnectedness between disorders, unifying them under the term "bipolar substance abuse." In three studies, IGT consistently produced better substance use outcomes even in comparison to a high-quality control intervention (i.e., group drug counseling).

3. What psychosocial intervention both focuses on the connections among thoughts, feelings, and behaviors and has strong evidence for benefit in treating people with mood disorders, SUDs, or both?

    A. Cognitive-behavioral therapy (CBT).
    B. Twelve-step facilitation.
    C. Motivational interviewing.
    D. Alcoholics Anonymous.

**The correct response is option A: Cognitive-behavioral therapy (CBT).**

CBT-based approaches to SUDs generally combine a focus on internal and external cues related to substance use (including distorted thinking) with enhancement of skills to manage risky interpersonal situations and psychological factors. CBT has perhaps the strongest evidence base supporting use in treatment of SUDs and co-occurring mood disorders. Not only does it have positive effects in reducing substance use or mood disorder symptoms when they occur as the sole diagnosis, it also has received significant study in those with co-occurring illnesses.

# Chapter 4

1. The best way to differentiate substance-induced anxiety disorder from a primary anxiety disorder is based on

    A. Duration of anxiety symptoms.
    B. Relationship of anxiety symptoms to periods of use or abstinence.
    C. Responsiveness to medications.
    D. Family history of anxiety disorder.

**The correct response is option B: Relationship of anxiety symptoms to periods of use or abstinence.**

The most reliable way to differentiate substance-induced anxiety disorder from primary anxiety disorder is to investigate whether there are enough diagnostic symptoms of anxiety during a prolonged period of abstinence. Cessation of anxiety during extended periods of abstinence suggests substance-induced anxiety disorder, whereas continued anxiety during periods of abstinence suggests primary anxiety disorder. Family history of anxiety disorder can increase likelihood of a primary anxiety disorder but is not sufficient for diagnosis. Duration of anxiety symptoms and responsiveness to medications are not helpful in this diagnostic clarification.

2.  Ms. G is a 42-year-old female who comes to your office with complaints of excessive alcohol use hindering her ability to maintain her job and stable interpersonal relationships as well as impairing social anxiety. You determine, based on the timeline of her symptoms, that her symptoms meet diagnostic criteria for social anxiety disorder and alcohol use disorder. She has never taken psychiatric medications before. Optimal initial treatment would include

    A. Disulfram and a selective serotonin reuptake inhibitor (SSRI).
    B. Trial of clonazepam and SSRI.
    C. Trial of an SSRI, naltrexone, and individual cognitive-behavioral therapy (CBT).
    D. Trial of SSRI, naltrexone, and a 12-step-based group abstinence program.

**The correct response is option C: Trial of an SSRI, naltrexone, and individual cognitive-behavioral therapy (CBT).**

Optimal treatment of a patient dually diagnosed with social anxiety disorder and alcohol use disorder (which frequently co-occur) would involve pharmacological and psychosocial treatments. A trial of a first-line medication for anxiety (usually an SSRI) along with pharmacological management of alcohol use disorder (with naltrexone or disulfiram) and psychotherapy would be recommended. However, group-based treatments are not efficacious in patients with social anxiety disorder and actually may increase anxiety, so individually based CBT would be recommended. Benzodiazepines are generally avoided in patients with substance use disorders because of their addictive potential.

3.  Which of the following medications should generally be avoided in a patient with both a primary anxiety disorder and an alcohol use disorder?

    A. Clonidine.
    B. Naltrexone.

    C. Lorazepam.
    D. Acamprosate.

**The correct response is option C: Lorazepam.**

Benzodiazepines are generally not recommended for treatment in the dually diagnosed patient because of their addictive potential. Additionally, bupropion is generally avoided because of concern for lowered seizure threshold, particularly in patients with alcohol or benzodiazepine use disorders.

# Chapter 5

1. Which of the following psychosocial approaches treats posttraumatic stress disorder (PTSD) and substance use disorders (SUDs) by addressing such topics as "Coping with Triggers" and "Self-Nurturing"?

    A. Alcoholics Anonymous.
    B. Biofeedback.
    C. Seeking Safety.
    D. Eye movement desensitization and reprocessing (EMDR).

**The correct response is option C: Seeking Safety.**

Seeking Safety is a structured, manualized therapy designed to reduce symptoms of co-occurring PTSD and SUDs by helping patients understand and explore the relationship between the disorders and teaching healthy coping skills for both. "Coping with Triggers" and "Self-Nurturing" are two of the 25 topics included in the manual.

2. Which of the following medications may be most effective for those individuals who develop PTSD prior to alcohol dependence?

    A. Sertraline.
    B. Naltrexone.
    C. Buprenorphine.
    D. Paroxetine.

**The correct response is option A: Sertraline.**

Studies by Brady et al. (2005) have shown that sertraline may be the most appropriate medication for those who develop PTSD prior to alcohol dependence.

3.  Which of the following is *true* about the evaluation of an individual with PTSD and a SUD?

    A.  A clinician can avoid questions about legal problems, because they are uncommon in individuals with PTSD and SUDs.
    B.  When an individual presents with symptoms of intoxication or withdrawal from a substance, he or she should not be immediately evaluated for PTSD.
    C.  Rarely are issues with smoking and smoking cessation encountered in individuals with PTSD and SUDs.
    D.  A clinician should focus, in the evaluation, on trauma that has occurred when individuals were not using substances.

**The correct response is option B: When an individual presents with symptoms of intoxication or withdrawal from a substance, he or she should not be immediately evaluated for PTSD.**

PTSD assessments should not be conducted until after patients are no longer in a state of intoxication or withdrawal. Veterans with comorbid PTSD and SUD have been shown to present with more symptoms of dependence, including a longer history of substance use, more social and legal problems, and more violent behaviors and suicide attempts. Individuals with PTSD who smoke are more likely to be heavy smokers and are less likely to quit smoking than those without PTSD. One theory as to why PTSD and SUDs commonly co-occur is because the states of hyperarousal that are associated with many intoxicated or withdrawal states put people at physiological risk for developing PTSD upon exposure to traumatic events.

# Chapter 6

1.  Which of the following psychosocial approaches has not had consistently strong evidence in decreasing substance use among patients with schizophrenia and substance use disorders?

    A.  Cognitive-behavioral therapy (CBT).
    B.  Dual Recovery Anonymous (aka "Double Trouble").

    C. Motivational enhancement therapy (MET).
    D. Contingency management.

**The correct response is option B: Dual Recovery Anonymous (aka "Double Trouble").**

While the 12-step model, as used in Dual Recovery Anonymous, may be useful in patients with strong spiritual backgrounds and high motivation, CBT, MET, and contingency management have strong evidence for reducing substance use outcomes.

2. Which medication used in patients with concurrent chronic psychotic illness and substance use disorder has been shown to be most effective in reducing substance use and increasing abstinence?

    A. Haloperidol.
    B. Olanzapine.
    C. Clozapine.
    D. Bupropion.

**The correct response is C: Clozapine.**

Although there is no good evidence for any benefit (and, in fact, even the suggestion of possible worsened substance use) from the use of first-generation antipsychotics in comorbid psychotic and substance use disorders, second-generation antipsychotics seem to play a role in decreasing cravings. Clozapine, in particular, has exceptionally impressive rates of decreased use of substances, increased abstinence, and fewer relapses. This may be due to clozapine's unique actions on serotonin and dopamine ($D_2$) receptors and the resulting effects in the dopamine reward pathways.

3. Which are the three most commonly used substances among patients with concurrent psychotic and substance use disorders?

    A. Alcohol, cocaine, marijuana.
    B. Alcohol, cocaine, nicotine.
    C. Cocaine, marijuana, nicotine.
    D. Alcohol, marijuana, nicotine.

**The correct response is option D: Alcohol, marijuana, nicotine.**

Nicotine, alcohol, and marijuana are the most commonly used substances among patients with schizophrenia, in that order. Cocaine is the next most frequently used substance.

# Chapter 7

1. Which of the following may make it difficult to diagnosis a personality disorder in an individual who is misusing substances?

    A. Few periods of abstinence.
    B. Late onset of substance use.
    C. Strong support system.
    D. Reliable historian.

    **The correct response is option A: Few periods of abstinence.**

    One reason that this effort is challenging is that an individual who uses one substance of abuse can appear wildly different when seen during withdrawal, during acute intoxication, and during persistent abuse. That same patient will look quite different while using a different substance or while using multiple substances. And that same person will think, feel, and behave differently after an extended period of sobriety. Since personality is defined as an enduring pattern of cognition, emotion, motivation, and behavior—and all of these are affected by substances—it can feel almost impossible to assess and potentially treat personality disorders in people with an active substance use disorder. Further, to diagnose a personality disorder, it is often helpful for the clinician to try to clarify personality disorders that might have existed prior to the onset of the substance abuse. This is complicated by the fact that substance abuse often starts during adolescence, when personality is still in formation, and by the reality that such data are retrospective and liable to error, even if collateral information is available.

2. Which of the following treatments has the most evidence for efficacy in individuals with borderline personality disorder (BPD) and substance use disorders?

    A. Medication management.
    B. Dialectical behavioral therapy (DBT).

    C. Psychodynamic psychotherapy.

    D. 12-step groups.

**The correct response is option B: Dialectical behavioral therapy (DBT).**

DBT has the most evidence for efficacy. This therapy involves individual and group modalities that combine standard cognitive-behavioral approaches with mindfulness, distress tolerance, and acceptance. Both regularly practiced DBT and modified DBT treatments that also explicitly address substance use have been shown to be helpful. DBT groups are now a component of most substance use treatment facilities.

3. Which of the following medications should be avoided or used with caution in an individual with BPD and a substance use disorder?

    A. Naltrexone.

    B. Lamotrigine.

    C. Lorazepam.

    D. Topiramate.

**The correct response is option C: Lorazepam.**

Benzodiazepines, although frequently prescribed for BPD, can lead to addiction and may actually be disinhibiting rather than calming.

# Chapter 8

1. A patient presents to you for treatment for cocaine use disorder. You conduct a structured interview, which confirms your suspicion of a diagnosis of attention-deficit/hyperactivity disorder (ADHD). Which of the following would be inaccurate in providing psychoeducation for the patient?

    A. "ADHD is very common in patients with substance use disorders. It's possible that part of why it's so difficult for you to quit on your own is because your ADHD symptoms are poorly managed."

    B. "Depression and anxiety are very uncommon symptoms when someone also has ADHD."

    C. "Patients with ADHD are sometimes not diagnosed during childhood, and some ADHD symptoms persist into adulthood."

    D. "Patients who use cocaine have similar rates of ADHD compared to individuals dependent on other drugs."

**The correct response is option B: "Depression and anxiety are very uncommon symptoms when someone also has ADHD."**

Comorbidity with other psychiatric disorders is very common.

2.   You initiate a trial of psychostimulant for an adolescent patient with comorbid ADHD and SUD. Her parents, however, have significant concerns that she might "get addicted" to the stimulant and sell the stimulant to her friends. Which of the following is incorrect and should not be included as part of your counseling for the family?

    A. "While psychostimulants carry a small risk of abuse, adequate treatment of ADHD is an important factor in successful control of the patient's substance use disorder."

    B. "While diversion is a concern for stimulants, especially in the college-age population, most college students who report using stimulants do so to study for exams or complete papers, rather than to get high."

    C. "While misuse of methylphenidate-based medications has been stable, misuse of prescription amphetamines has been dramatically increasing."

    D. "Longer-acting formulations of psychostimulant generally have a lower liability for misuse compared with immediate-release formulations."

**The correct response is option C: "While misuse of methylphenidate-based medications has been stable, misuse of prescription amphetamines has been dramatically increasing."**

Misuse of prescription amphetamines has stayed relatively stable over the past decade. All the other items are true.

3.   Your patient, who has both an alcohol use disorder and a cocaine use disorder, received initial treatment with a long-acting methylphenidate preparation for his ADHD. His symptoms of ADHD improved but did not fully remit, and he continues to use cocaine sporadically, though he has stopped drinking. Which of the following is *true* for revising his treatment plan?

A. Higher-than-standard dosing of mixed-amphetamine salts may reduce both ADHD and substance use.
B. Atomoxetine is generally ineffective for treating ADHD symptoms in adults with alcohol use disorder.
C. Amphetamines, as opposed to methylphenidate, have been found to increase cocaine use in patients with both alcohol and cocaine use disorders, and are therefore contraindicated in this patient.
D. Cognitive-behavioral therapy (CBT) produces a minimal reduction in ADHD symptoms.

**The correct response is option A: Higher-than-standard dosing of mixed-amphetamine salts may reduce both ADHD and substance use.**

Higher-than-standard dosing of mixed-amphetamine salts can reduce both ADHD and substance use. Atomoxetine has been shown to be effective in reducing ADHD symptoms. Amphetamine formulations do not increase cocaine use. CBT is effective in reducing ADHD symptoms.

# Chapter 9

1. Which of the following contributes to the high prevalence of tobacco abuse in eating disorders (EDs)?

   A. Tobacco is notorious for suppressing appetite.
   B. Advertising for cigarettes has historically been associated with excessive eating.
   C. Smoking is more commonly seen in the restricting type of EDs.
   D. Tobacco use is associated with eating solid foods in social settings.

**The correct response is option A: Tobacco is notorious for suppressing appetite.**

Tobacco is notorious for suppressing appetite. Advertising for cigarettes has historically catered to a cultural drive for "thinness." Though nicotine is often associated with weight loss, statistics show that smoking is more prevalent in binge-purge patients who also show net weight *gains* over time. Cigarette abuse is heavily associated with symptoms of mood dysregulation and impulsivity, which are often comorbid in bulimia nervosa (BN) and binge-eating disorder. Cigarette smoking provides an alternative activity to eating solid food in social settings.

2.  Which medication is commonly used in the management of substance use disorders (SUDs) but may be contraindicated in anorexia nervosa (AN)?

   A. Topiramate.
   B. Bupropion.
   C. Naltrexone.
   D. Citalopram.

**The correct response is option B: Bupropion.**

Bupropion is a first-line medication for smoking cessation and can be quite effective in curbing substance cravings. It can also function as a useful alternative to selective serotonin reuptake inhibitors (SSRIs) or tricyclic antidepressants when the depressive and amotivational features tied to substance abuse are a focus of treatment. Despite these positive attributes, its use in treating low-weight patients is relatively contraindicated because there is a significant risk of seizures (the combination of medication and malnutrition can significantly lower one's seizure threshold). Of note, patients with AN may request this medication despite its side effects, since it is also known to be an effective appetite suppressant.

3.  Which one of the following evidence-based psychotherapy approaches would be most ideal when first approaching a 31-year-old patient who is of low to average weight, purging multiple days per week, and struggling with intermittent heroin abuse?

   A. Psychodynamic psychotherapy, followed by antidepressant trial.
   B. Motivational interviewing, followed by a trial of cognitive-behavioral therapy (CBT) or dialectical behavioral therapy (DBT).
   C. Family-based treatment (FBT) alone.
   D. 12-step group program for BN.

**The correct response is option B: Motivational interviewing, followed by a trial of cognitive-behavioral therapy (CBT) or dialectical behavioral therapy (DBT).**

Though there is no clear standard-bearer when it comes to acute management of comorbid EDs and SUDs, the initial use of motivational interviewing to ascertain the patient's willingness to commit to an evidence-based psychotherapy is recommended, followed by a course of CBT or DBT (both of which have emerging support in the literature as a primary treatment). The addition of an SSRI trial while receiving psychotherapy would also be indicated; however, there is much less support for the use of psychodynamic psychotherapy over behavioral approaches. The use of FBT would apply more to children and teens with the restricting type of AN (parents assume a structured feeding program at home). It may be useful to augment treatment with a 12-step program such as Alcoholics Anonymous or Overeaters Anonymous, though monotherapy with this approach would not be preferable.

# Chapter 10

1. Approximately what percentage of individuals with gambling disorder (GD) has any lifetime comorbid substance use disorder (SUD)?

    A. 5%–10%.
    B. 20%–30%.
    C. 40%–60%.
    D. More than 60%.

**The correct response is option D: More than 60%.**

According to the largest epidemiological study conducted in the United States, by Petry and colleagues, among respondents with GD, the lifetime prevalence rates of any alcohol and drug use disorder were 73% and 38%, respectively.

2. Which of the following is *true* regarding the comorbidity between GD and SUD?

A. Patients with co-occurring GD and SUD have better clinical outcomes compared with those without a SUD.

B. Alcohol consumption paired with gambling is associated with smaller average bets and less money lost.

C. Withdrawal symptoms and tolerance are characteristic of SUDs and GD.

D. The prevalence of other psychiatric disorders, such as mood, anxiety, or personality disorders, is significantly lower in individuals with both GD and SUD than in individuals with only GD.

**The correct response is option C: Withdrawal symptoms and tolerance are characteristic of SUDs and GD.**

GD and SUD share several phenomenological characteristics (e.g., loss of control, urges, persistent/recurrent behavior despite its serious negative consequences). Symptoms characterizing both SUD and GD also include withdrawal symptoms (restlessness or irritability when attempting to cut down/stop gambling) and tolerance (betting increasing amounts of money).

3.   Which of the following psychotherapeutic treatments is the most efficacious in the treatment of GD?

A. Assertive community treatment (ACT).

B. Cognitive-behavioral therapy (CBT).

C. Contingency management.

D. Dialectical behavioral therapy (DBT).

**The correct response is option B: Cognitive-behavioral therapy (CBT).**

CBT has the strongest evidence of efficacy in GD. CBT focuses on achieving abstinence from gambling by helping patients acquire specific skills that enable lifestyle changes and restructure the environment to increase reinforcement from non-gambling behaviors. ACT and DBT are not evidence-based treatments for gambling disorders (nor is psychodynamic psychotherapy). Contingency management treatment utilizes rewards (e.g., prizes) to reinforce positive behaviors (e.g., abstinence) and has been proven effective in clinical trials on several SUDs. Even though studies suggest that prize-based contingency management does not increase gambling, its use is controversial in GD given that some prize-based incentives have an element of chance that may be considered similar to gambling.

# Chapter 11

1.  How many members does Alcoholics Anonymous (AA) have?

    A. 100,000.
    B. 500,000.
    C. 1 million.
    D. 2 million+.

    **The correct response is option D: 2 million+.**

    Alcoholics Anonymous is a mutual-aid fellowship started in 1935 by Bill Wilson and Dr. Bob Smith. For at least 100 years prior to the founding of AA, other grassroots efforts to address alcoholism emerged but ultimately failed. AA now counts over 2 million members with more than 115,000 registered groups.

2.  Which of the following is *true* about AA or Narcotics Anonymous (NA)?

    A. AA was the first mutual aid fellowship to encourage abstinence from alcohol in its members.
    B. A belief in God is an essential component of NA.
    C. Most 12-step programs discourage members from taking psychiatric medications.
    D. The only requirement for AA membership is a desire to stop drinking.

    **The correct response is option D: The only requirement for AA membership is a desire to stop drinking.**

    As indicated in the 12 traditions, the only requirement for AA membership is a desire to stop drinking. AA was the most successful, but not the first, grassroots effort to address alcoholism. A belief in a higher power is an important component of 12-step programs; the second step states, "Came to believe a Power greater than ourselves could restore us to sanity." However, the higher power is defined by the individual, and a belief in God is not a requirement for membership in NA (or AA). A survey of 12-step representatives indicate that the majority feel that individuals with mental illness should continue taking their medication. Significant paranoia may interfere with 12-step attendance but is not an absolute contraindication.

3. Which of the following is *true* regarding 12-step participation and individuals with co-occurring disorders (CODs)?

    A. Twelve-step participation rates in individuals with CODs are generally comparable to those in individuals with substance use disorders (SUDs) only.
    B. Individuals with CODs are more likely to be referred to 12-step programs than are those with SUDs only.
    C. Individuals with CODs attending Double Trouble in Recovery (DTR) have lower rates of abstinence than individuals attending AA with substance use disorders only.
    D. A major disadvantage of 12-step programs is cost.

**The correct response is option A: Twelve-step participation rates in individuals with CODs are generally comparable to those in individuals with substance use disorders (SUDs) only.**

Research on 12-step attendance and effectiveness in individuals with CODs is limited, and there is minimal evidence comparing the efficacy of DTR with that of other 12-step programs for individuals without CODs. However, most of the available data suggest that 12-step participation rates are comparable for individuals with CODs despite being underutilized. A major advantage of 12-step programs is cost.

# Chapter 12

1. The first process in motivational interviewing (MI) is

    A. Assessment.
    B. Screening.
    C. Engaging.
    D. Planning.

**The correct response is option C: Engaging.**

The first process of MI is engaging. To begin the process of change, the therapist needs to form a positive therapeutic alliance with the client, in large part by accurately understanding, without casting judgment, the client's perspective and demonstrating compassion and acceptance toward the client.

2. The specific problem focus of MI treatment is determined by which of the following?

   A. Therapist.
   B. Client.
   C. Referral source.
   D. Client's past history.

**The correct response is option B: Client.**

The specific problem focus of treatment for dually diagnosed clients is based on the client's goals and preferences. Therapists guide the process of bringing focus to a problem area, but they ultimately respect the client's choice and priorities as a starting point for motivational enhancement.

3. Which of the following should be avoided when using MI with individuals with co-occurring disorders?

   A. Targeting medication and treatment program adherence in addition to substance use.
   B. Using successive reflections and summaries.
   C. Incorporating concrete and engaging methods for eliciting change talk.
   D. Discussing complex psychodynamic formulations.

**The correct response is option D: Discussing complex psychodynamic formulations.**

When the therapist is working with a client who has severe psychiatric symptoms and substance use problems, it is helpful to address adherence to treatment, including medications; frequently use successive reflections and summaries to help accommodate the client's psychiatric symptoms and cognitive limitations; and incorporate concrete and engaging methods to hold the client's attention and bring emphasis to his or her motivations for change.

# Chapter 13

1. Which of the following best describes a "gold standard" dual diagnosis inpatient unit?

   A. An inpatient detoxification unit with direct linkage to an inpatient psychiatry unit.
   B. An inpatient unit staffed by internists and psychiatrists in order to provide complete medical and psychiatric care.
   C. An inpatient unit employing motivation enhancement therapy, relapse prevention, contingency management, and 12-step group work.
   D. An inpatient unit with a focus on transitioning patients to long-term residential treatment upon discharge.

   **The correct response is option C: An inpatient unit employing motivation enhancement therapy, relapse prevention, contingency management, and 12-step group work.**

   Although the concept of a "gold standard" dual diagnosis unit is not set in stone, option C comes closest to describing what has been proposed in this chapter as optimal. Essentially, it is a psychiatric inpatient unit with significant treatment for substance use disorders woven into the daily functioning of the unit, including motivational interviewing/enhancement therapy techniques, relapse prevention, contingency management, and 12-step group work. Although options A, B, and D describe units that would benefit those with a substance use disorder, they are not part of our definition here.

2. Based on the proposed taxonomy of addiction treatment programs discussed in this chapter and the ASAM patient placement criteria, an acutely suicidal patient at risk of alcohol withdrawal should be matched to which of the following treatment settings:

   A. Level III, Inpatient, medically monitored, Dual diagnosis enhanced.
   B. Level III, Residential, Addiction only services.
   C. Level IV, Inpatient medically managed, Dual diagnosis enhanced.
   D. Level III, Residential, Dual diagnosis capable.

**The correct response is option C: Level IV, Inpatient medically managed, Dual diagnosis enhanced.**

Dually diagnosed patients with severe or debilitating psychiatric illness (e.g., entailing risk of self-harm or unable to tend to self care) who are at risk of imminent and life-threatening withdrawal require medically intensive inpatient treatment services (ASAM Level IV) in a dual diagnosis enhanced unit. This involves 24-hour medical and nursing care typically rendered in an acute psychiatric unit by staff credentialed in evidence-based mental health and substance abuse treatment. Dual diagnosis capable (DDC) facilities represent a less intensive level of care suitable for patients with stable psychiatric comorbidities that do not interfere with participation in substance abuse treatment. ASAM Level III encompasses treatment levels from clinically managed low-intensity residential services (nonmedical or social detoxification) to medically monitored high-intensity inpatient services (such as free-standing detoxification centers) but is inappropriate for patients at acute risk of self harm or life-endangering withdrawal.

3. Which of the following factors may limit the efficacy of traditional 12-step programs as recovery resource for the dually diagnosed and lead to underutilization of mutual help services?

    A. Confrontation as a therapeutic strategy.
    B. Illness-related factors such as cognitive impairment and paranoia.
    C. An "anti-prescription" bias.
    D. All of the above.

**The correct response is option D: All of the above.**

Traditional 12-step programs are important and effective recovery resources for patients with substance use disorders. The dually diagnosed, however, face unique challenges that may bear significantly on their ability to benefit from such programs. Aspects of traditional 12-step fellowships such as confrontational therapeutic strategies and bias against prescription medications (including psychotropics) may discourage attendance and participation or lead to noncompliance and decompensation among the dually diagnosed. Illness-related factors such as paranoia or social anxiety may further inhibit involvement in 12-step programs and impair recovery outcomes for the dually diagnosed. Specialized mutual-help programs such as Double Trouble in Recovery have emerged to address these limitations of traditional 12-step programs.

4.  Which of the following forms of treatment discussed in this chapter have been found to increase the likelihood of showing up to the first postdischarge appointment?

    A. Cognitive-behavioral therapy.
    B. Motivational interviewing.
    C. Art therapy.
    D. Psychodynamic psychotherapy.

**The correct response is option B: Motivational interviewing.**

Both motivational interviewing and music therapy have been associated with increasing the likelihood of showing up to the first post-discharge appointment. In a recent randomized controlled trial, by Pantalon and colleagues, dually diagnosed men were at least 9.5 times more likely to show up to the first postdischarge appointment as an outpatient if they received brief motivational interviewing while hospitalized. In a pilot study, by Ross and colleagues, taking place on a dual diagnosis unit, the number of music therapy sessions attended appeared to be linked to a greater likelihood of showing up to the aftercare appointment even after the study authors controlled for length of stay.

# Chapter 14

1.  Approximately what percentage of individuals with substance use disorders (SUDs) receive pharmacological treatment for their SUD?

    A. 10%.
    B. 25%.
    C. 50%.
    D. 75%.

**The correct response is option A: 10%.**

While individuals with CODs often receive treatment for their psychiatric disorders, very few end up receiving treatment for their

SUDs. This may be especially problematic for individuals with opioid use disorder. Starting opioid agonist therapy after an overdose, for example, has been associated with a 50% reduction in subsequent death, yet less than 5% of those who survive an overdose receive pharmacotherapy.

2.  Which of the following medications may treat both an individual's personality disorder and his or her SUD?

    A. Gabapentin.
    B. Topiramate.
    C. Disulfiram.
    D. Naltrexone.

**The correct response is option B: Topiramate.**

Topiramate has evidence for treating alcohol use disorder and borderline personality disorder. Although gabapentin may treat alcohol use disorder and help treat anxiety and mood states, there is little evidence that it can treat personality disorders. Disulfiram and naltrexone are primarily used to treat SUDs.

3.  Which of the following is a contraindication to starting naltrexone?

    A. Current depressive episode.
    B. Renal impairment.
    C. Severe liver failure.
    D. Current treatment with escitalopram.

**The correct response is option C: Severe liver failure.**

In general, naltrexone can be easily combined with psychotropic medications without concern for interactions or neuropsychiatric side effects. Contraindications include acute hepatitis or severe liver disease.

# Chapter 15

1.  A 15-year-old patient presents to the emergency room in a post-ictal state after a witnessed seizure with a urine toxicology positive for benzodiazepines. The first step in management is

    A. Refer to an outpatient clinic for a substance abuse evaluation.

    B. Call parents and provide them with a list of 12-step groups in the area that are geared toward adolescents and young adults.

    C. Admit to the neurology service for epilepsy workup.

    D. Observe in emergency department, checking vital signs frequently, and attempt to obtain collateral history from parents and/or peers.

**The correct response is option D: Observe in emergency department, checking vital signs frequently, and attempt to obtain collateral history from parents and/or peers.**

The first step in developing a treatment plan for an adolescent with substance use is to address safety. This patient, who may be actively intoxicated and/or in active withdrawal from a benzodiazepine, must be stabilized medically before any further treatment recommendations can be made. Referral to an outpatient evaluation or to a 12-step group may be appropriate in the future (options A and B), when the patient is stabilized and further history is obtained and he appears to have an active substance use problem. However, the immediate concern is to manage further withdrawal from the benzodiazepine in a medically safe manner. Admission to the neurology service for an epilepsy workup is premature, given that the patient has had only one seizure, in the presence of benzodiazepine in the urine (option C). Option D is most appropriate, because by monitoring the patient's vital signs and overall medical status in the emergency department, withdrawal can be managed while further history is obtained from others and eventually from the patient himself, when he is no longer in a post-ictal state.

2.   Which of the following is a primary reason adolescence is a developmentally vulnerable period with regard to the development of substance use problems?

    A. The brain continues to develop until the mid-twenties.

    B. The "top-down" controls provided by the prefrontal cortex cannot be overruled by the "bottom-up" force of the reward system in adolescents.

    C. The risk-avoidance mechanism of the amygdala cannot be overridden by the reward-seeking mechanism of the ventral striatum.

D. The adolescent brain has more opioid receptors than the adult brain because they have not yet been fully pruned.

**The correct response is option A: The brain continues to develop until the mid-twenties.**

The adolescent brain indeed continues to develop until the mid-twenties, with top down and risk-avoidance mechanisms developing later than reward-seeking mechanisms (options A, B, and C). There is not evidence that opioid receptors are more abundant in the adolescent brain than they are in the adult brain, let alone because of pruning, which usually refers to synapses rather than receptors.

3. The following approach is best for maintaining an adolescent's request for confidentiality while also maintaining her safety with regard to substance use:

A. Advise the adolescent that if she does not disclose her use to the parent, the clinician will do so.
B. Advise the adolescent that confidentiality will be maintained, no matter what, so the adolescent should feel secure sharing anything with the clinician.
C. Advise the adolescent that engaging her parents in treatment will make it most effective, such that some information that the adolescent discloses to the clinician may be metabolized into treatment recommendations that are given to the parents.
D. Advise the adolescent that confidentiality will only be breached if safety becomes an issue, and that any substance use behaviors in an adolescent are inherently unsafe.

**The correct response is option C: Advise the adolescent that engaging her parents in treatment will make it most effective, such that some information that the adolescent discloses to the clinician may be metabolized into treatment recommendations that are given to the parents.**

Helping adolescents to feel secure in disclosing information about their substance use, without over-promising unconditional confidentiality, is a special challenge in adolescent substance use treatment. Threats or coercion (option A), are not usually effective and tend to undermine treatment alliance with adolescents. Option B would be inappropriate, since confidentiality will always be breached if acute safety is an issue. Option D is inappropriate in that substance use is not by definition a safety issue in adolescents, and such an extreme stance will discourage open discussion. Option C is reasonable, because even though the clinician can usually avoid disclosing specific details to parents, parents will need to have a general understanding of the problem at hand to the extent necessary for the clinician to provide treatment recommendations.

# Chapter 16

1. Which of the following statements is *true* regarding substance use disorders (SUDs) in older adults?

    A. Demographic trends suggest a decreasing prevalence of SUDs in older adults in the coming decade.
    B. Older men have not been shown to have higher rates of alcohol and psychoactive substance problems when compared with older women.
    C. Overall alcohol use increases with age.
    D. Older adults who engage in treatment have worse adherence when compared with their younger counterparts.

    **The correct response is option B: Older men have not been shown to have higher rates of alcohol and psychoactive substance problems when compared with older women.**

    Older men have been shown to have higher rates of alcohol problems than older women but lower rates of prescribed psychoactive substance misuse when compared with older women. Demographic trends suggest an increasing prevalence of SUDs in older adults in the coming decade. Alcohol use decreases with age. Older adults who engage in treatment have better adherence when compared with their younger counterparts.

2. Which of the following statements is *true* regarding the diagnosis of SUDs in older adults?

    A. SUDs in older adults are underdetected and underdiagnosed.
    B. With age, referrals for treatment of SUDs are less likely to come from primary care settings and more likely to come from the criminal justice system.

    C. Guidelines recommend the same level of alcohol consump-
       tion in older adults and the same thresholds to diagnose prob-
       lematic drinking.
    D. There are no validated screening tools for alcohol use disorder
       that have been specifically adapted for the geriatric population.

**The correct response is option A: SUDs in older adults are under-
detected and underdiagnosed.**

SUDs in older adults are underdetected and underdiagnosed in part
because the presenting features can mimic common medical, neurological, and psychiatric disorders. With age, referrals for treatment of SUDs are more likely to come from primary care settings
and less likely to come from the criminal justice system. As a result
of age-related vulnerabilities, guidelines recommend lower alcohol
consumption in older adults and lower thresholds to diagnose problematic drinking. The Michigan Alcoholism Screening Test—Geriatric Version (MAST-G), and its abbreviated version (SMAST-G), have
been adapted for and validated in older adults.

3.   Which of the following characteristics of treatment for SUDs are pos-
    itively correlated with engagement and response in older adults?

    A. Mixed-age treatment and specialty care setting.
    B. Age-specific treatment and specialty care setting.
    C. Mixed-age treatment and integrated care setting.
    D. Age-specific treatment and integrated care setting.

**The correct response is option D: Age-specific treatment and inte-
grated care setting.**

Age-specific treatment and an integrated care model have been
shown to improve treatment adherence and outcomes in older adults.

# Chapter 17

1.   A transgender male patient who has been taking testosterone by in-
    tramuscular means for several years now has developed crystal meth
    addiction and has been known to inject or "slam" the drug. In your
    treatment, what should you suggest about testosterone?

A. Advise him to stop testosterone. It is likely leading to the crystal meth addiction.
B. Look for other forms of testosterone treatment. Injecting the medication may be a trigger.
C. Continue intramuscular testosterone. There is no need for further assessment when providing trans-affirming care.
D. Consider that he is abusing testosterone in addition to crystal meth.

**The correct response is option B: Look for other forms of testosterone treatment. Injecting the medication may be a trigger.**

It is important to be mindful of triggers in a patient's recovery. Although testosterone has no influence on the patient's sobriety, the act of injecting the drug could be a trigger. Consider other forms of testosterone for continued care.

2. A young cisgender teenager who recently started to explore his sexual feelings discovered that he is attracted to other boys and has tried to keep it a secret from his family and friends because of their strict religious associations. He started using alcohol with his friends and was noticed to drink large amounts and have blackouts. He was taken to the emergency room one night because his parents noticed him recently having mood swings and they discovered he has been telling friends at school he is thinking about suicide. What should be the first steps with this patient?

A. Think about prescribing a mood stabilizer. He may be suffering from bipolar disorder and a medication like lithium could prevent suicide.
B. Refer him to reparative therapy. If a therapist can help him have feelings toward girls, his suicidality will resolve.
C. Arrange a family meeting to clarify the patient's homosexuality.
D. Create a safety plan around suicide and start LGBTQ-affirming care. Allow him to discuss his feelings in an open and nonjudgmental environment.

**The correct response is option D: Create a safety plan around suicide and start LGBTQ-affirming care. Allow him to discuss his feelings in an open and nonjudgmental environment.**

Safety comes first with suicidal patients. Once a plan around safety has been made, the most supportive and appropriate treatment would be LGBTQ-affirmative care. Confronting the parents may put more stress on the patient and medication should be avoided unless the patient does not respond to basic supportive interventions. Reparative therapy could do more harm to the patient and lead to suicide.

3. A 35-year-old cisgender gay man comes to an outpatient clinic with crystal meth addiction. He uses crystal meth when he is sexually active, and this causes him to have intense hallucinations and paranoia. He recently lost his job and is facing homelessness due to the addiction. Which is the best possible treatment available to this patient?

    A. Crystal Meth Anonymous.
    B. Abstinence program.
    C. Antipsychotic medication.
    D. Stimulants.
    E. Motivational interviewing.
    F. Group therapy.
    G. Selective serotonin reuptake inhibitors.
    H. All of the above.

**The correct response is option H: All of the above.**

All these are acceptable forms of treatment for the symptoms listed. The treatment chosen should depend on the patient's clinical presentation and what kind of treatment they desire. Keep all possible options on the table when evaluating a new patient and be open to different pathways to sobriety.

# Chapter 18

1. According to the Bureau of Justice Statistics, what percentage of incarcerated individuals with mental illness reported being under the influence of a substance at the time of their offense?

    A. >25%.
    B. >33%.
    C. >50%.
    D. 0%.

**The correct response is option B: >33%.**

According to a 2006 report from the Bureau of Justice Statistics, over a third of incarcerated patients were using substances at the time of their alleged crime.

2.  Which of the following is a difference between a prison and a jail?

    A. Average duration of incarceration.
    B. There are no differences between the two.
    C. Prisons hold more dangerous criminals.
    D. Treatment is more challenging in prisons because inmates do not have a known discharge date.

**The correct response is option A: Average duration of incarceration.**

*Jails* are short-term facilities that house people who have been newly arrested, sentenced to less than a year, or are awaiting disposition of their criminal cases. Sixty percent of jail inmates have not been convicted of a crime and are awaiting action on their criminal cases. Because they do not have a known discharge date, treatment planning can be difficult. *Prisons* are longer-term facilities that house sentenced inmates. There are no distinctions between jails and prisons regarding dangerousness of the inmate population.

3.  Which of following is *true* about diversion programs?

    A. Most drug and mental health courts do not offer treatment with agonist medications.
    B. Drug and mental health courts do not reduce illicit drug use and recidivism and fail to improve adherence to treatment.
    C. Most communities have failed to keep diversion programs in operation without federal funding.
    D. Inmates cannot be diverted for mental illness prior to arraignment.

**The correct response is option A: Most drug and mental health courts do not offer treatment with agonist medications.**

In the United States, diversion programs have become increasingly popular as a means of diverting nonviolent offenders away from jails and prisons into more treatment-oriented settings. While 98% of diversion programs report opioid-addicted participants, only 47% offer agonist medication (56% offer medication-assisted treatment, which includes the opiate antagonist naltrexone). According to a 2006 survey on drug use and health from the Department of Health, diverted individuals drink less frequently (59% alcohol users at baseline compared with 28% at 6-month follow-up), use less alcohol (38% drinking to intoxication at baseline compared with 13% at 6-month follow-up), and use fewer drugs (58% at baseline compared with 17% at 6-month follow-up). When the 12 months following participation in an alternative to the incarceration program were compared with the preceding 12 months, participants had fewer arrests (2.3 vs. 1.1), and spent fewer days in jail (52 vs. 35) following diversion. These courts often exclude violent offenders on the basis of current or past criminal charges. Three of four jail diversion programs keep operating after federal funding ends.

# Index

*Page numbers printed in **boldface** type refer to tables and figures.*